more
smoothies *for* life

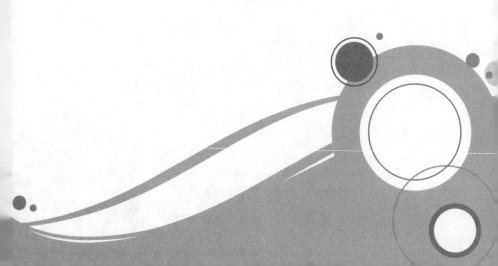

OTHER BOOKS BY DANIELLA CHACE

Smoothies for Life

The New Detox Diet
with Elson M. Haas

What to Eat if You Have Cancer
with Maureen Keane

The What to Eat if You Have Cancer Cookbook
with Maureen Keane

What to Eat if You Have Diabetes

The What to Eat if You Have Diabetes Cookbook

What to Eat if You Have Heart Disease
with Maureen Keane

The What to Eat if You Have Heart Disease Cookbook

Pressure-Cooking the Easy Way
with Maureen Keane

Pressure-Cooking the Meatless Way
with Maureen Keane

The Ultimate Pressure-Cooker Cookbook
with Maureen Keane

Bread Machine Baking for Better Health
with Maureen Keane

The RV Cookbook
with Amy Boyer

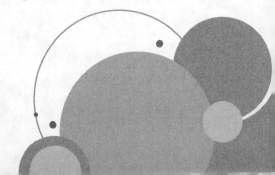

more
smoothies *for* life

satisfy, energize
& heal your body

• • •

Daniella Chace

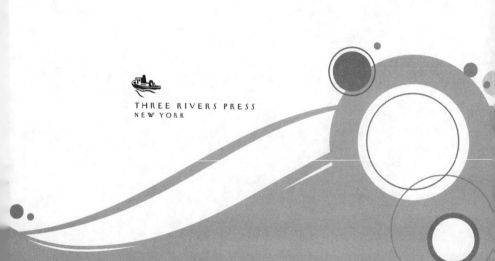

THREE RIVERS PRESS
NEW YORK

Copyright © 2007 by Daniella Chace

Published in the United States by Three Rivers Press, an imprint of the
Crown Publishing Group, a division of Random House, Inc., New York.
www.crownpublishing.com

Three Rivers Press and the Tugboat design are registered trademarks of
Random House, Inc.

Library of Congress Cataloging-in-Publication Data

Chace, Daniella.
    More smoothies for life : satisfy, energize, and heal your body / Daniella Chace.
        p. cm.
    Includes index.
    1. Fruit drinks.   2. Smoothies (Beverages).   I. Title.
    TX815.C44 2007
    641.8'75—dc22   2007002861

ISBN 978-0-307-35136-4

Printed in the United States of America

Design by Nora Rosansky

10 9 8 7 6 5 4 3 2 1

First Edition

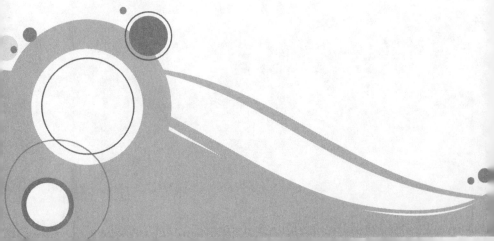

I dedicate this book to my life-long mentor in whole-foods creations, the lovely and clever Linda Kay Landkammer, who continues to inspire me in making "food as medicine" in delicious ways. I love you, Mom!

I also want to give my editor, Brandi Bowles, a very sincere thank-you for her attention to detail and dedication to the scientific aspects of medicinal smoothie creations.

I appreciate my recipe-development teams and thank them for all of their experimentation and exploration, and for sharing with us their delicious discoveries.

All of the recipes in this book have been analyzed using Esha Research, Inc., software, which is widely recognized as one of the leading nutritional analysis programs in the industry. Their expansive database has allowed us to bring you the most accurate nutrient breakdown possible for each of the smoothie recipes in this book.

And finally it is with huge gratitude that I acknowledge my assistant Tara Hubbard, who reigns supreme as the driver of the Esha Software in my office!

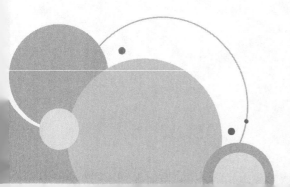

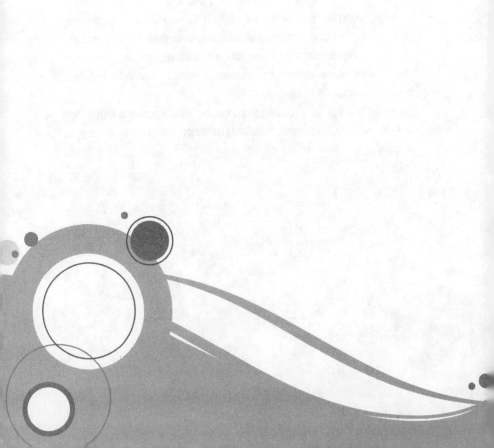

acknowledgments

Bellevue, Washington

Tony and Katie Chace, who have traveled the world looking for the best smoothies and found their favorites in Hawaii, for the hours of recipe testing in the Hailey test kitchen. Mike Ristow, the Blender Barrista of Bellevue, for assisting in the creation of numerous smoothie recipes. Julie Mermelstein, my childhood partner in messy kitchen creations. Ray and Darleen Horton, for their patience as I learned how to use a blender at age thirteen. Thanks for cleaning up the chocolate from every kitchen surface after my blender-blunder all those years ago.

Kona, Hawaii

Linda Landkammer, for spending several weeks in a condo in Kona, creating and tasting endless, scrumptious recipes with me. Hunter Brooks, for his guidance into the world of tropical fruit and for the many hours of research, fact checking, and editing. Shane Balucan, James Cram, Paulette Spence, and their cohorts for the local lore about Hawaiian culture; history of medicinal plants, herbs, fruits, and berries; and culinary tips. "Mango Mike" Oros, on Maui, for his tips on locating the best smoothie ingredients and for being my mango expert. Una Greenway and Leon Rosner, of Kuaiwi Farm in Captain Cook, Hawaii, and Joan and Tom Lamont, of Happy Honu Farm, for the Saturday Market education.

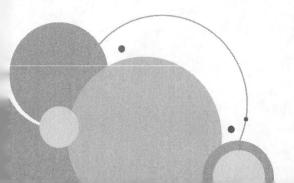

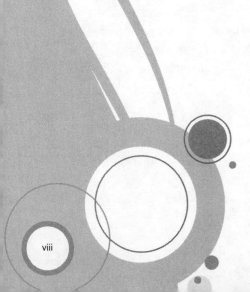

Hailey, Idaho

Alysson Heazle, for her kitchen assistance and recipe testing until we had the ratios "just right," and to her darling bambinos—Ms. Riley Revallier, for her contribution of the Bubbly Fruit Cooler from summer camp (which she says is "super good") and her thirteen-month-old brother, Noah, our recipe tester for the baby recipes. Noah tasted all of the baby recipes and gave us either a head shake and furrowed brow or a big smile. Kassie Knopp, for the Mexican Chocolate creation. Cygnia Rapp, of Organic Prosperity Foods, for the medical studies on coconut oil and flax oil. Adam King, Lori Nakaoka, Elana King-Nakaoka, Sara King-Nakaoka, and their friend Kari Zamora, my family of testers who developed some of the most exotic concoctions in the book.

And finally, to Gary Boyer, my most dedicated smoothie taster, who not only tasted about a hundred recipes but also drank blenders full of them so we didn't waste a drop.

contents

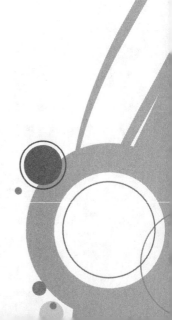

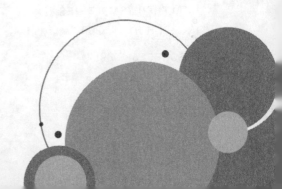

more
smoothies *for* life

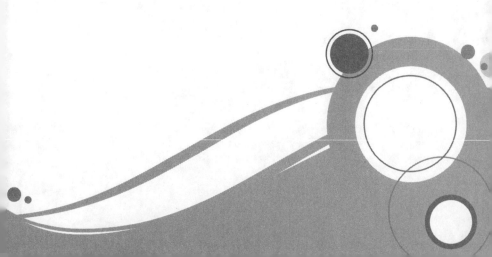

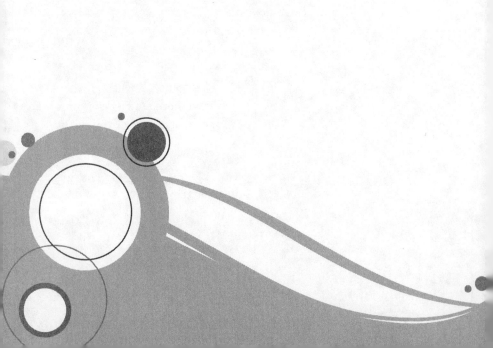

introduction

It's a well-known fact that Americans don't get enough fruits and vegetables. Health experts have been warning us about this deficiency for nearly fifty years, but we're so used to hearing admonishments about our health that we often gloss over them without reflection. However, the fact remains that if you fail to get the recommended amounts of the essential nutrients you need every day, you will face the consequences. Nutrient deficiencies caused by poor diet manifest in lowered immune function, high blood pressure, premature graying of the hair, brittle nails, slowed metabolism, higher risk for heart disease and cancer, and—gasp!—rapid aging. The point of this reminder isn't to scare you, but to get you thinking about the big picture and shrug off the casual indifference that is ruining our country's health.

The only person who's going to impact your health and longevity is *you*, and it'll come by being open-minded, experimental, and well informed. Luckily, there's no better time to start eating right than right now, as we are in the middle of the most rapidly evolving time in the history of food science. Every week new studies are published, such as those touting the health benefits of whole foods, and resources like this book take the most relevant information from these studies and distill it into wholesome, everyday recipes that can pluck you right out of the declining status quo!

Nutrients Are Color, Color Is Nutrients!

One of the most fascinating discoveries of recent food science has been the fact that we can see certain nutrients as color in foods. The pigments in living things such as plants, algae, and animals are actually compounds that perform a variety of biological functions for us. For example, one well-known group of pigments are the carotenoids, which include nutrients such as beta-carotene. Carotenoids give fruits and vegetables their yellow, orange, and green color; they act as antioxidants, protect our skin from chemicals and the sun's rays, and provide the body with the components to make vitamin A on demand. Pretty cool, right?! And all it takes to replenish your body with these important nutrients is to remember to eat lots of green, yellow, and orange foods.

The New World—of Food Science Discoveries

There is a plethora of newly discovered phytochemicals, or naturally occurring plant chemicals, in fruits and vegetables. Studies are being conducted right now that identify specific phytochemicals and the diseases that they alter. Sometimes they are found to help prevent a disease and other times they can be used as a treatment. Quite often they are found to be more effective than pharmaceutical agents in reducing the symptoms of a health condition or disease.

Some of the nutrients recently identified are flavonoids, which are found in blueberries, blackberries, and citrus fruits. These strengthen cell membranes, help prevent bruising, and have powerful disease-fighting benefits.

Natural Chemicals That Fight Disease

Flavonoids are not mysterious substances seen only with a microscope. They are polyphenolic chemicals that give foods color, texture, and taste. You can actually see and taste them. This is true for many of the nutrients in fruits and vegetables. Four thousand flavonoids have been discovered so far and more are being researched as we speak.

Flavanones such as hesperetin, naringenin, and eriodictyol are found in citrus fruits such as oranges, lemons, and grapefruits. They play a major role in the prevention of heart disease. Flavones such as luteolin and apigenin are antioxidants that also protect the heart and vascular system, promote healthy blood sugar levels, and reduce inflammation. Apigenin is a flavone found in peppermint and chamomile that has antioxidant, anti-tumor, and anti-inflammatory properties.

Catechins such as proanthocyanidins are a type of antioxidant found in chocolate, apples, apricots, cherries, peaches, raspberries, strawberries, and blackberries, as well as green and black teas. Catechins help protect us because they are free-radical scavengers that also promote vascular relaxation and help prevent atherosclerosis (hardening of the arteries).

Another subclass of flavonoids is anthocyanins, which impart the violet, blue, and purple colors that we see in fruits, berries, and flowers. The violet anthocyanins give color to black currants, purple grapes, blueberries, blackberries, and plums. Red anthocyanins are present in red berries such as lingonberries, cranberries, red currants, and cherries. Eating this group of flavonoid-rich foods can help reduce your risk of developing coronary heart disease (CHD) by reducing the production of LDL (bad) cholesterol.

Serious Medicine Never Tasted So Good

Pomegranates have been a popular fruit in the Middle East, Spain, and Italy for centuries. Now that we see the health benefits of the juice of this fruit, we are starting to incorporate it into our diets as well. Promising new studies brought pomegranates into the spotlight when it was discovered that drinking just one glass of pomegranate juice every day for one year reduces blood pressure and the oxidation that causes the "bad" LDL cholesterol to stick to the artery walls. Food scientists credit the pomegranate's tannins, polyphenols, and anthocyanins for these particular cardiovascular benefits. Best of all, this is one of the richest-tasting fruit juices out there.

A specific component of pomegranate juice, called ellagic acid, was found to be protective against several types of cancer. One particularly impressive study from the University of South Carolina's Hollings Cancer Institute found that ellagic acid stops cancer cells from dividing in patients with breast, pancreas, esophageal, skin, colon, and prostate cancers. An equally exciting study from Japan found that when leukemia patients drank pomegranate extracts, leukemia cells reverted to their normal noncancerous state.

Even the common apple is getting a little more respect in the medical world these days. A recent study found that rats fed the equivalent of one to six apples per day developed fewer breast-cancer tumors, even after being treated with a carcinogen known to trigger mammary cancer. The average apple, it turns out, is a rich source of the flavonoid quercetin, which protects our cells from cancer and our blood vessels from chemical damage—once again proving that old adages often have validity and our grandmothers were right.

Population studies are generating an impressive number of new reports on the reduction of disease risk for those who drink tea. Any tea will do, it appears, as each has its own health-generating properties. Green and black teas contain natural phytochemicals called polyphenols, which have cardiovascular protecting effects, and white tea is very high in antioxidants.

Studies that look at groups of people with specific dietary habits are helpful in showing us the potential benefits of a particular food. For example, the National Cancer Institute found that Chinese men and women who drank green tea had a whopping 60 percent reduced risk of esophageal cancer.

One medicinal food that Americans are more than willing to incorporate into their diets is cocoa. I'd like to take a minute now to pay homage to this delight, befitting our palates. I'd also like to give thanks to the researchers at the University of California in San Francisco who discovered its medicinal benefits so that we can partake with pride. Numerous studies have confirmed that cocoa is a rich source of antioxidant flavonoids with beneficial cardiovascular properties such as vasodilatation and blood pressure reduction, inhibition of platelet activity, and decreased inflammation. The caveat is that to get these benefits, you must eat it daily. They recommend about 1.6 ounces per day—now that's a prescription I can live with!

Nutrient Powerhouse in a Glass

With so much research behind the medical efficacy of a wide variety of smoothie-worthy fruits, I find I can easily justify taking a few minutes out of my day to whip up an elixir of tasty ingredients that have so many concrete health benefits.

Having the information you need to choose the ingredients that address your health concerns gives you the medicinal and culinary tools to become a nutrition wizard in your own kitchen. The next step is to organize a tasting party for yourself or your family. It's important that you learn which flavors and textures you love, so that you will be more likely to make smoothies a part of your health program for the long run.

Your daily smoothie can give you a tremendous health advantage by rejuvenating, healing, and preventing disease for you, every single day.

If you have a hard time swallowing a lot of supplements, it's very simple to open some of them up and pour them right into your drink. You may also find foods that are rich in the nutrients you have been taking in supplement form, which may reduce your supplement load. For example, if you take electrolytes, fiber, antioxidants, protein, and minerals, you can create a daily drink similar to the Strawberry-Blueberry Ginger recipe (see page 32) and never have to worry about those supplements again.

Imbibing a delicious, creamy drink daily can be good medicine. You can literally reverse nutrient deficiencies, slow down the oxidative processes (aging) of your cells, make your nails stronger and your hair shiny, protect yourself from heart disease and cancer, and provide your body with the nutrients it needs to have more energy and boost your metabolism (fat burning). Now, that's a dessert you deserve.

Let's get started. Practice your nutritional wizardry and get creative in your kitchen. Go bananas, have fun, get healthy!

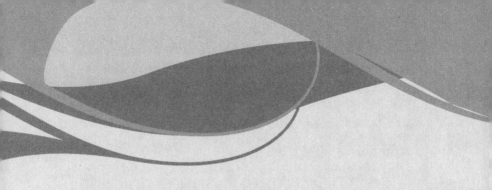

...The Basics...

Be Your Own Nutritionist

Smoothies are so personal. These creamy or sparkling concoctions are made of ingredients chosen by you, tailored to your personal taste, with the nutrients you need to feel vital and full of energy. If you arm yourself with the knowledge of basic nutrition, you can be your own nutritionist and personal chef, and indulge in a bit of healthy hedonism every day with cumulative health benefits.

Blend Like a Pro

The learning curve for becoming a blender pro with skills to brag about is not too steep. After playing around with just a few recipes, you will quickly get a feel for how to create your preferred texture with either frozen fruit or ice. Then you can concentrate on developing the flavors that really make you smile. Maybe you'll lean toward the cool and refreshing, with sparkling water and lemon juice; or perhaps it will be the more lush, milk-based drinks with sweet fruit like peaches that most tickle your palate. As you gain experience through experiments, one day, perhaps unintentionally, you will mix the perfect combination of ingredients—the smoothie that makes you squeal with delight. Then you'll be hooked and ready to share your talents with your world.

A Smoothie a Day

I fell in love with smoothies while working as a nutritionist in clinical practice. They seemed to be the answer for many of my clients' nutritional deficiencies. Most of my clients were busy, active people with substantial protein and electrolyte needs, yet by the very nature of their lifestyles they had a hard time finding time in the day to plan, prepare, and eat meals.

I started to play in my kitchen to create nutritionally potent smoothies that met my clients' particular needs. I found that many of them weren't getting enough protein, which left them feeling tired and craving sugar, so I would often start with a protein base in their smoothie. I developed the following list to help them choose high-protein foods that fit their palates. They would then add to the mix any supplements they were already taking. For example, probiotics taste like whey and easily blend in smoothies, thus eliminating a daily capsule. I also discovered that electrolytes blend well in citrus drinks, and that liquid multivitamins are virtually undetectable in fruit purees. Here are the approximate protein values for some common smoothie ingredients.

PROTEIN FOODS FOR SMOOTHIES		
PORTION SIZE	FOOD	PROTEIN
½ cup	Cottage cheese, 1% fat	14 grams
1 cup	Low-fat plain yogurt	12 grams
3 ounces	Extra-firm tofu	10 grams
4½ ounces	Firm tofu	10 grams
6 ounces	Soft tofu	10 grams
7½ ounces	Silken tofu	10 grams

PORTION SIZE	FOOD	PROTEIN
¼ cup	Sunflower seeds	10 grams
¼ cup	Pumpkin seeds	8.5 grams
1 cup	Skim, 1%, 2%, whole milk, and buttermilk	8 grams
1 cup	Soymilk	8 grams
1 tablespoon	Peanut butter	4 grams
1 tablespoon	Soy butter	4 grams
1 tablespoon	Sunflower butter	3 grams
1 tablespoon	Cashew butter	2.8 grams
1 tablespoon	Tahini (sesame butter)	2.6 grams
1 tablespoon	Almond butter	2.4 grams
1 tablespoon	Hazelnut butter	2 grams
1 tablespoon	Nonfat dry milk	1.5 grams

Smoothies for Life—*The Sequel*

When I wrote *Smoothies for Life* with Maureen Keane in 1998, we designed the book to meet many of the country's most prevalent nutrition-related health concerns at that time. Unsurprisingly, many of the same conditions are still hot topics today. People still seek to increase their energy, enhance their libido, detoxify, burn body fat, and increase muscle mass. The response to the first book was phenomenal, and many people reported positive results from our healthful recipes. However, the pace of nutrition science has grown exponentially since then, giving us exciting new discoveries that have now been incorporated in this sequel.

Functional Natural Foods

Thousands of new medical nutrition studies that are published every year provide us with information about what I call "functional natural foods." I am referring specifically to foods that help us treat many health conditions. This used to involve some guesswork and often a fair bit of folklore, but we now know of numerous nutrients that have proven effective in healing disease and increasing health. For example, the antioxidant-rich Amazonian fruit açaí (pronounced *ah*-SIGH-*yee*) is all the rage in smoothie bars, and for good reason. Açaí juice is used to protect our bodies from environmental toxins. Mangosteen is enjoying huge popularity, as medical studies appear monthly in the journals regarding its neuroprotective, anti-inflammatory, and antihistamine effects. Similarly, pomegranate is in the spotlight as numerous studies are taking a closer look at its cancer-defying phytochemicals.

Delicious Medicine

In this book, I have translated these food-science studies into groupings of foods that support specific health conditions so you can make medicinally active smoothies that meet your specific health needs. In addition, by making smoothies at home, you control the quality of the ingredients you use. You may use decaf coffee for your coffee-based drinks, for instance, or all organic ingredients, if you so choose. You may want to order an especially hard-to-find ingredient that supports your health and use it daily in your drinks, just as you would take your daily multi-vitamin capsule. Think of this book as an open resource or guide to making the best culinary decisions for your life.

In each chapter, I have translated studies relating to disease and diet, and culled out the nutrients used to affect that condition. I have also created a food list that contains the nutrients most appropriate for smoothies. For example, vitamin C is found in tangerines, oranges, kiwi, strawberries, potatoes, cabbage, and red peppers, but if you put the latter three in a blender, I'm blameless for the results.

How to Make Smoothies

To get started all you need is a blender. Food processors and hand-held blenders work well, too. A classic smoothie recipe contains liquid, fruit, and either ice or frozen fruit.

Basic Smoothie

1 cup liquid
1 frozen fruit

Start with a liquid base such as fruit juice or milk, then add fruit. It's that simple. Frozen fruit will give your drink a creamy texture and cool sensation. To puree chunks of raw fruit, place them in a blender with a small amount of liquid until you have reached the preferred consistency. Then add the remaining ingredients. Smoothies are one of my favorite foods to make because there aren't any hard-and-fast rules. Use ice to cool your drinks if you want to cut calories or increase your water intake. Add fresh or frozen fruit in myriad combinations. Add protein sources such as peanut butter, yogurt, or nonfat dry milk for energy—these all add great texture as well. Once you discover your favorite flavor combinations, you can begin to perfect the textures with bulkier additions, such as wheat germ, granola, or more frozen fruit. To personalize your drinks you can add your favorite protein sources and supplements that you may already be taking, or you can add new supplements such as electrolyte powder, vitamin C powder, or probiotics. The final touch is in the presentation. Stacking thick, cold drinks in tall glasses with a slice of fruit as a garnish or serving ice-cold drinks in glass tumblers are easy ways to tantalize yourself or your guests and greatly enhance your sipping experience. Who knew healthy living could be this much fun?

Smoothie Terminology

For the sake of simplicity, I have abbreviated generic terms such as *milk*. When a recipe calls for milk, you can use the milk of your choice, such as soy, dairy, nut, or grain milks. "Sparkling water" refers to mineral waters such as San Pellegrino and Perrier. These natural mineral waters are often sold in glass bottles to avoid the unhealthy contaminants that can be leached from plastic. Always buy products carbonated with CO_2 and avoid products carbonated with phosphorous or phosphoric acid. Although using phosphorus is a much more common method for carbonating water and soda, it can interfere with mineral metabolism.

Another term you may not be familiar with yet, because I just made it up, is *frapoothie*. I thought we needed a word to describe a blended coffee drink with fruits and other nutritional elements. But mostly I just really like the word because it's so ridiculous that it makes me laugh. If Starbucks can coin the term *Frappuccino* by combining the Italian cappuccino with the Greek frappé, I don't see why we can't all make up our own terms and copyright them or register them. So if you come up with a wacky and wonderful combination, claim the patent and then include its name in your vocabulary. You never know who might be listening in.

I like how well these terms describe the texture of a drink. Although they all refer to smoothies, some are smoother than others.

SMOOTHIE TEXTURE TERMINOLOGY

Cooler — Cold, light, and refreshing; generally juice-based rather than cream-based.

Frappé — Icy blend with milk froth.

Frapoothie — Blended coffee drink with fruits and other nutritional elements.

Freeze — Thick, cold, ice-based drink.

Frosty — Similar to a freeze.

Icy — Cold with ice crystals, not smooth.

Shake — Cream-based, cold, rich, and flavorful.

Smoothie — Creamy and cold, generally with frozen fruit rather than ice.

Whip — Light and frothy.

Smoothie Ingredients Defined

Sparkling water: This refers to naturally carbonated mineral water such as Perrier, San Pellegrino, and San Faustino.

Cocoa powder: I use organic, unsweetened, dark cocoa powder for its low sugar content and high antioxidant levels.

Ice: Taste the ice first to be sure it doesn't contain chlorine, which can ruin a smoothie. Use a filter on your automatic ice-maker or fill your ice trays with filtered water to avoid chlorine and other contaminants. If you don't have a filter, you can leave chlorinated water out overnight and the chlorine will evaporate from the water.

Milk: The term *milk* refers to all milk products and milk alternatives, such as whole dairy milk, reduced-fat dairy milk, almond milk, soymilk, rice milk, or oat milk. In every case, it is strongly recommended that you buy organic. Nonorganic dairy is often contaminated with agricultural chemicals and bovine growth hormone. Ninety-five percent of nonorganic soy is genetically engineered to have a higher resistance to herbicides. This means higher chemical-residue levels on the beans and lower nutritional value. Recent studies found that the medicinal benefits were dramatically reduced in GMO (genetically modified organism) soybeans.

Protein powder: Protein powder supplements come from many sources, such as rice, soybeans, dairy, or peas. Some powder compounds also include vitamins, minerals, or herbs, and many are flavored. Plain or vanilla provide the most versatility when making smoothies. Choose the source based on your own sensitivities or flavor preference. When using powders, pour the liquid in first and then the powder, otherwise it will tend to stick to the inside of the blender.

Supplements: Vitamins, minerals, amino acids, probiotics, antioxidants, and other nutrients can be added to smoothies. If they are in capsules, you'll need to open them first and then pour the contents into your drink. It's wise to taste them first to be sure they won't destroy the flavor of your smoothie.

Sweeteners: Choose your sweeteners not only by flavor but also for their caloric content and other nutritional benefits. Xylitol, for example, is the kind of sweetener that works well for iced-tea–type drinks, but also helps encourage the colonization of microflora, whereas most sweeteners offer only small quantities of minerals at best. Xylitol, stevia, and the chicory-based Just Like Sugar™ are good for diabetics, as they do not raise blood sugar levels. Stevia works well in heavier shakes that hide its flavor a bit.

Avoid all synthetic sweeteners such as aspartame, sucralose, and saccharin. Animal and human studies have repeatedly proven their negative effects. Natural sweeteners like honey, brown rice syrup, real maple syrup, agave, dried malt, and barley malt syrup are all fine additions to smoothies, and each adds its own unique flavor. Also, when reading ingredient lists, be aware that many words ending in *-ose* (such as sucrose, glucose, fructose, and dextrose) are forms of sugar. The benefit of eating whole organic foods is that you can often avoid excessive and unhealthy sugars and decide for yourself what sweeteners will go in your body.

Thickeners: Frozen fruit and ice will give smoothies body, but nothing helps control texture and consistency like healthy thickening agents. These are added to help emulsify ingredients, so they won't separate as quickly after blending. They include psyllium powder, ground flaxseed, and reconstituted gelatin.

FRUIT LIST

Açaí	Blueberries
Apples, peeled and pitted	Cantaloupe, rind removed
Applesauce	Cherries, pitted
Apricots, peeled and pitted	Cranberries
Avocados, peeled and pitted	Cucumber, peeled
Bananas, peeled	Currants
Blackberries	Dates, pitted

Figs, chopped
Gooseberries
Grapefruit, peeled and
   seeded
Grapes, seedless
Guava
Honeydew melon, rind
   removed
Huckleberries
Kiwis, peeled
Kumquats
Lemons, seeded and peeled
Limes, peeled and seeded
Loganberries
Lychee, peeled and pitted
Mangoes, peeled and pitted
Marionberries
Nectarines, peeled and
   pitted

Oranges, peeled and seeded
Papayas, peeled and pitted
Passionfruit, peeled
Peaches, peeled and pitted
Pears, peeled and cored
Persimmons, peeled
Pineapples, peeled and cored
Plums, peeled and pitted
Pomegranate, seeds only
Prunes, pitted
Pumpkin, peeled and seeded
Raisins
Raspberries
Star fruit
Strawberries
Tangerines, peeled and
   seeded
Watermelon, seeded and
   rind removed

LIQUIDS LIST

Amazake
Apple juice
Coffee
Dairy milk
   Chocolate milk
   Goat's milk
   Kefir
   Lactose-free milk
   1%, 2%, and whole milk
   Yogurt
Fruit juice
Fruit sauces
Grain milk
   Mixed grain milk
   Oat milk
   Rice milk
Herbal tea
Ices

Nectars
   Coconut
   Guava
   Mango
Nut and seed milk
   Almond milk
   Coconut milk
   Hazelnut milk
   Sesame seed milk
Soymilk
   Whole, low-fat, plain or
   flavored
Sparkling water
Tea (green or black)
Vegetable juice
   Beet
   Carrot
   Tomato
Water, filtered

Basic Kitchen Tools

Blenders

Buying a blender: Look for blenders with sharp blades, a glass pitcher rather than plastic, and a strong motor.

Using an old blender: If you have an old blender with dull blades or a wimpy motor, consider those traits when preparing your ingredients. You may want to cut up your fruit a bit smaller and use smaller portions of ice. Be sure you have enough liquid so that the motor doesn't have to strain against a thick mixture of ingredients. In addition, you may have to peek in more frequently to be sure that food has not packed around the blades. If this happens, turn the blender off, use a spatula to dislodge the food or ice, then continue to blend.

Blender assembly: Before you get started, be sure that the rubber ring is in place between the pitcher base and the cutting assembly. It is easy to forget to put the rubber ring back in after you have taken everything apart to wash the blender. I forgot the ring once, and lost so much of my smoothie out the bottom of the pitcher that I'll never make the same mistake again.

Blender lid: Always cover the blender before you start to blend. At thirteen, I attempted a chocolate concoction at a friend's house and made the mistake of turning on the blender without the lid in place. Her parents found splats of chocolate on every surface imaginable for at least the next three months.

Utensils

Spatulas: Heat-resistant spatulas hold up better and are made of healthier materials. Buy narrow, long-handled spatulas that can easily reach the bottom of the blender and fit around the blades.

Knives: A sharp chef's knife and a paring knife are helpful. They are safer than regular kitchen knives as they slice into foods more easily, thus reducing the chance that they will slip off of a round fruit and into your finger. You can have your knives sharpened professionally or hone them yourself on the bottom of a ceramic mug to give them a crisp edge. When using sharp knives, always cut round fruits in half and place the flat side down so they aren't rolling as you're cutting.

Spoons: Use long-handled spoons that can reach down into the space near the blades. Be sure to turn off the blender *before* using any utensils near the blades.

Cutting boards: Use a different cutting board for your smoothie ingredients from the one you use for meats. Raw meat can contaminate the board with toxic bacteria. If you use a wood cutting board, sand it down periodically to remove the deep grooves that may harbor bacteria. Use hot water and dish soap to wash your boards after every use. Run them through the dishwasher for a deeper cleansing.

Preparation and Storage

If you don't have time to run to the store every time you want to whip up your favorite smoothie, you may want to buy mass quantities of your favorite ingredients and store them so you're ready for a healthy treat at a moment's notice.

Bulk: Buy foods that do not need refrigeration and last for months on the shelf. If you purchase your favorite items by the case, most grocers will give you a discount. Freezer items will last for months, too. Most milks are available in aseptic boxes, which don't need refrigeration until they're opened.

Glass: Glass bottles are safer than plastics, as chemicals in plastics can interfere with the hormones in our bodies, and do not leach chemicals, such as bisphenol A, into the liquid you drink.

Pantry: Fruit and vegetable juice, purees, sauces, and slices in glass containers will last for a year until they are opened. Bottled water, nut butters, dried fruits, aseptic boxes of tofu, and many other packaged foods can be stored in quantity in the pantry, which means fewer trips to the store.

Fridge: Keep perishables refrigerated, and buy only foods that you will use in the next week.

Freezer: Keep a bag of ice or a full ice tray on hand if you don't have an icemaker. Frozen concentrates, frozen fruit in bags, and protein powders can be stored for months in the freezer. If you have access to fresh fruit, you may want to pick your own and then freeze it. This is often an economical choice for ripe fruit in season such as mangoes, bananas, and berries. If you're freezing berries you have picked and washed, be sure to let them dry out before freezing so they don't clump in the freezer bag; otherwise it's hard to get just the quantity you want when it's time to use them. One technique is to pat them dry with a clean towel and then freeze them individually by spreading them out on a baking sheet. Place them in the freezer for about 2 hours to harden before you pour them into a freezer bag. They will then keep for about a year, especially if you have used double-thickness ziplock bags. When fresh produce is not available, try to buy fruits and vegetables that are frozen when ripe. These often have higher nutrient levels than produce that has been shipped long distances.

Freezing bananas: Peel them first, then break them into chunks and throw them into ziplock bags for freezing.

Now that you have done your homework, you know almost everything you need to create the ultimate personalized smoothie. In the following pages, you'll be introduced to a number of smoothie recipes, food studies, and suggestions for getting the most out of your daily shake. You're well on your way to whipping up a cool tall one—a gift to yourself for taking such fantastic care of your own body. It literally is its own reward.

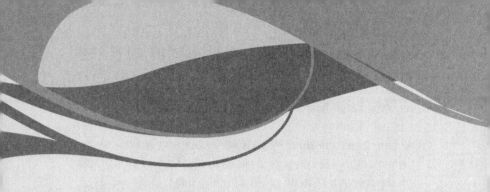

...Wellness...

There are several simple nutritional strategies to improve your general health and vitality. First, hydrate! This doctrine is so simple and yet so often overlooked. Boost your protein intake. Protein from plant sources is full of amino acids that support thousands of biological processes. By eating plant protein rather than animal protein, you are automatically taking in fiber. Plant foods also contain antioxidants and other phyto-chemicals that support health and healing.

General Nutrition Guidelines

Hydration

Keeping ourselves hydrated is one of the simplest and yet most important steps we can take to stay well. Consider the following:

- Lack of water is the primary cause of daytime fatigue and headaches.
- 50 percent of Americans are chronically dehydrated.
- In 37 percent of Americans, the thirst mechanism is so weak that it is often mistaken for hunger. Even mild dehydration will slow down one's metabolism by as much as 3 percent, and severe dehydration by 5 percent.

- One glass of water shut down midnight hunger pangs for almost all of the dieters studied in a University of Washington study.
- Preliminary research indicates that 8 to 10 glasses of water a day could significantly ease back and joint pain for up to 80 percent of sufferers.
- A mere 2 percent drop in body water can trigger fuzzy short-term memory, trouble with basic math, and difficulty focusing on the computer screen or on a printed page.

> ## HOW MUCH WATER SHOULD YOU DRINK?
>
> Take your weight and divide it in half to get the number of ounces of water you need per day, as a baseline. For example, a 120-pound person needs a minimum of 60 ounces of water a day.

Protein

Along with carbohydrates and fat, protein is one of the three macro-nutrients we need for good health. Adequate protein intake throughout our lifetime facilitates the growth, repair, and maintenance of every cell in our bodies. Infants and children require more protein per pound of body weight than adults, since the early years are a time of constant growth and development.

When we eat foods that contain protein, our digestive system breaks it down into amino acids, which are in turn used by our bodies for a multitude of tasks. Protein facilitates water balance, is a source of heat and energy, helps maintain a healthy acid-base balance, assists with disease resistance and cell repair, aids in maintaining blood sugar levels, and is necessary for building and maintaining lean body mass.

How much protein do we need? The recommended intake of protein is generally about 15 to 25 percent of your total caloric intake. Age, gender, and body weight determine an individual's caloric needs, and protein needs are calculated as a percentage of total calories consumed each day. Following is a chart that lists protein needs based on caloric intake.

PROTEIN NEEDS BASED ON DAILY CALORIC INTAKE	
1,200 calories/day	45 to 75 grams protein
1,500 calories/day	56 to 93 grams protein
2,000 calories/day	75 to 125 grams protein
2,500 calories/day	93 to 156 grams protein
3,000 calories/day	112 to 187 grams protein

Fairly sedentary people need only .36 grams of protein per pound of body weight. (Infants, children, athletes, and pregnant and nursing women require more.) To calculate the exact amount you need, multiply your ideal weight by .36. This will give you your optimum daily protein requirement in grams.

What are the best sources of protein? Meeting our protein needs from a variety of sources, with an emphasis on whole foods (foods that are organically grown and have undergone minimal processing), is an ideal strategy; this way you cover all of your vitamin and nutrient needs as well. Integrating new plant-based protein foods into your diet can have a host of positive benefits, and you may even discover a whole new array of foods that are not only healthful but tasty, too!

Fiber

Soluble and insoluble fiber are important to our diets because they help clean up the digestive tract and bind with harmful toxins to help eliminate them. Fruits, vegetables, and whole grains are all sources of fiber. To add more fiber to smoothies, add cooked grains such as brown rice, quinoa, or oatmeal; add whole fruit that is fresh, frozen, pureed, or dried; or add cooked vegetables such as carrots, beets, or greens to your smoothies.

Antioxidants

There is a tremendous amount of research regarding antioxidant activity in foods now. To help us choose the real superstars, government scientists have released this list of the twenty foods with the highest concentrations of natural antioxidants. These numbers reflect the total antioxidant capacity (TAC) per serving (1 piece fruit/potato, ½ cup beans/dried fruit, 1 cup berries/artichoke hearts, 1 ounce nuts).

ANTIOXIDANT-PACKED FOODS TAC	
Small red beans	13,727
Wild blueberries	13,427
Kidney beans (red)	13,259
Pinto beans	11,864
Cultivated blueberries	9,019
Cranberries	8,983
Artichokes	7,904
Blackberries	7,701
Dried plums (prunes)	7,291
Raspberries	6,058
Strawberries	5,938
Red Delicious apple	5,900
Granny Smith apple	5,381
Pecans	5,095
Sweet cherries	4,873
Black plums	4,844
Russet potato	4,649
Black beans	4,181
Plums	4,118
Gala apple	3,903
Walnuts	3,846

Cocoa Smoothie

Dates are an absolutely delicious sweetener for smoothies. They are a good fiber source and have a subtle flavor that doesn't compete with other ingredients.

1 cup soymilk
3 tablespoons unsweetened cocoa powder
3 dates, pitted
1 ripe banana, peeled

Serves 1

Look for organic cocoa powder, such as Dagoba Organic Chocolate cocoa powders.

Cocoa is naturally rich in antioxidant polyphenols that fight the free radicals that damage body tissue.

SERVING SIZE: 1 (449G)			
CALORIES: 490		**CALORIES FROM FAT: 60**	
	%DV*		%DV*
Total Fat 7g	11%	Sugars 69g	
Saturated Fat .5g	3%	Protein 17g	
Cholesterol 0mg	0%	Vitamin A	4%
Sodium 105mg	4%	Vitamin C	15%
Total Carbohydrate 104g	35%	Calcium	15%
Dietary Fiber 12g	48%	Iron	20%
*Percent Daily Values are based on a 2,000 calorie diet			

Guava Slurpee

Tropical fruit juice bottled with its fiber has become known as nectar. Many nectars are sold in glass bottles and are available in grocery stores.

1 cup guava nectar
1 cup ice cubes
1 cup strawberries, hulled
½ cup yogurt

Serves 1

Adding yogurt to your daily smoothies ensures your intake of protein, calcium, and microflora.

SERVING SIZE: 1 (827G)			
CALORIES: 290		**CALORIES FROM FAT: 10**	
	%DV*		%DV*
Total Fat 1g	2%	Sugars 56g	
Saturated Fat 0g	0%	Protein 9g	
Cholesterol 5mg	2%	Vitamin A	15%
Sodium 130mg	5%	Vitamin C	300%
Total Carbohydrate 65g	22%	Calcium	25%
Dietary Fiber 6g	24%	Iron	6%
* Percent Daily Values are based on a 2,000 calorie diet			

Cherry Parfait

Even though this tastes like a dessert, it's actually a nutrient-dense drink that makes an excellent breakfast.

1 cup milk
1 cup yogurt
1 cup pitted cherries
½ cup granola

Serves 2

Cherries (both fresh and frozen) contain the flavanoid quercetin, which helps combat heart disease, cataracts, allergies, inflammation, bronchitis, and asthma.

> Japanese researchers reported that 80 percent of people who ate 8 ounces of natural yogurt daily for six weeks had a decrease in sulfide compounds, the odoriferous chemicals responsible for halitosis.

SERVING SIZE: ½ OF RECIPE (320G)			
CALORIES: 250		**CALORIES FROM FAT: 60**	
	%DV*		%DV*
Total Fat 7g	11%	Sugars 25g	
Saturated Fat 2.5g	13%	Protein 14g	
Cholesterol 15mg	5%	Vitamin A	10%
Sodium 170mg	7%	Vitamin C	4%
Total Carbohydrate 36g	12%	Calcium	35%
Dietary Fiber 3g	12%	Iron	2%
*Percent Daily Values are based on a 2,000 calorie diet			

Breakfast Blend

This classic combination is a favorite daily smoothie to support the immune system.

1 cup milk
½ cup orange juice
1 frozen peeled banana
¼ cup cottage cheese
1 teaspoon sweetener

Serves 1

Even if you don't love cottage cheese, try it in smoothies. It's high in protein and low in calories, and so creamy that it's hard to detect once blended.

SERVING SIZE: 1 (550G)			
CALORIES: 380		**CALORIES FROM FAT: 100**	
	%DV*		%DV*
Total Fat 11g	17%	Sugars 43g	
Saturated Fat 6g	30%	Protein 17g	
Cholesterol 30mg	10%	Vitamin A	15%
Sodium 300mg	13%	Vitamin C	120%
Total Carbohydrate 59g	20%	Calcium	35%
Dietary Fiber 3g	12%	Iron	4%
*Percent Daily Values are based on a 2,000 calorie diet			

Pumpkin Pie Smoothie

Canned pumpkin puree is often overlooked as a smoothie ingredient, yet it's a dreamy addition. The texture is like pudding and makes for a very satisfying and filling shake.

1 cup pumpkin puree
½ cup ice cubes
½ cup evaporated milk
¼ cup orange juice
2 tablespoons sweetener
½ teaspoon grated nutmeg
½ teaspoon ground cinnamon

Serves 2

Cinnamon's ability to reduce blood sugar and cholesterol levels has been well established in the medical research. Those prone to high blood pressure or high cholesterol may want to include cinnamon in their daily smoothie. The pumpkin is packed full of carotenoids and fiber.

SERVING SIZE: ½ OF RECIPE (293G)			
CALORIES: 210		**CALORIES FROM FAT: 45**	
	%DV*		%DV*
Total Fat 5g	8%	Sugars 29g	
Saturated Fat 3g	15%	Protein 6g	
Cholesterol 20mg	7%	Vitamin A	350%
Sodium 70mg	3%	Vitamin C	25%
Total Carbohydrate 36g	12%	Calcium	20%
Dietary Fiber 5g	20%	Iron	6%
*Percent Daily Values are based on a 2,000 calorie diet			

mon-Lime Punch

Garnish this snappy concoction with a fresh mint leaf and a lime or lemon wedge.

½ cup apple juice
½ cup sparkling water
1 tablespoon lime juice
1 tablespoon fresh lemon juice
1 teaspoon electrolyte powder

Serves 1

This refreshing drink is a good hydrator, as it contains fructose, water, and electrolytes.

SERVING SIZE: 1 (277G)			
CALORIES: 60		**CALORIES FROM FAT: 0**	
	%DV*		%DV*
Total Fat 0g	0%	Sugars 14g	
Saturated Fat 0g	0%	Protein 0g	
Cholesterol 0mg	0%	Vitamin A	0%
Sodium 0mg	0%	Vitamin C	20%
Total Carbohydrate 17g	6%	Calcium	10%
Dietary Fiber 0g	0%	Iron	2%
*Percent Daily Values are based on a 2,000 calorie diet			

Ruby Orange Icy

The Sicilian red orange, also called the blood orange because of its ruby red flesh, is rich in the powerful antioxidant anthocyanin, which gives the orange its red pigment.

1 cup fresh orange juice
1 orange, peeled, sectioned, and frozen
Optional: ½ cup ice cubes
¼ teaspoon vanilla extract

Serves 1

Keep frozen orange segments on hand for a quick icy. Peel oranges and break into sections, then toss them in a ziplock freezer bag and freeze them for future use.

Blood oranges are now widely available and are excellent sources of vitamin C, potassium, and fiber, especially if you use the whole orange in your smoothies. In fact, one medium orange provides 28 percent of the recommended daily intake for dietary fiber.

SERVING SIZE: 1 (402G)			
CALORIES: 190		**CALORIES FROM FAT: 5**	
	%DV*		%DV*
Total Fat 0g	0%	Sugars 35g	
Saturated Fat 0g	0%	Protein 3g	
Cholesterol 0mg	0%	Vitamin A	10%
Sodium 0mg	0%	Vitamin C	340%
Total Carbohydrate 47g	16%	Calcium	8%
Dietary Fiber 7g	28%	Iron	4%
*Percent Daily Values are based on a 2,000 calorie diet			

Tropical Sunrise

Frozen bananas give smoothies a thick and creamy texture. This fruity combination is like a sweet sorbet.

1 mango, peeled and pitted
1 frozen peeled banana
½ cup nectar (guava, mango, coconut, etc.)
½ cup pineapple chunks

Serves 1

Tropical fruit provide vitamin C, fiber, antioxidant carotenoids, and natural fruit sugars that support immune function and overall wellness.

SERVING SIZE: 1 (499G)			
CALORIES: 330		**CALORIES FROM FAT: 10**	
	%DV*		%DV*
Total Fat 1g	2%	Sugars 67g	
Saturated Fat 0g	0%	Protein 3g	
Cholesterol 0mg	0%	Vitamin A	45%
Sodium 10mg	0%	Vitamin C	140%
Total Carbohydrate 86g	29%	Calcium	6%
Dietary Fiber 8g	32%	Iron	6%
*Percent Daily Values are based on a 2,000 calorie diet			

Blueberry Tea

This drink is as bright, vivid, and healthful as it is tasty, and it makes for a great afternoon pick-me-up.

1 cup green tea
1 cup blueberry juice
½ cup blueberries
½ cup ice cubes
1 teaspoon electrolyte powder

Serves 1

Blueberry juice and green tea combine to form a potent elixir of antioxidants that offer the heart and all the cells protection from environmental toxins.

> Catechins, which are antioxidants found in fresh tea leaves, appear in concentrations of up to 30 percent of dry weight for white and green tea leaves, but black tea has substantially less owing to its oxidative preparation.

SERVING SIZE: 1 (685G)			
CALORIES: 180		**CALORIES FROM FAT: 0**	
	%DV*		%DV*
Total Fat 0g	0%	Sugars 31g	
Saturated Fat 0g	0%	Protein 2g	
Cholesterol 0mg	0%	Vitamin A	0%
Sodium 50mg	2%	Vitamin C	10%
Total Carbohydrate 45g	15%	Calcium	15%
Dietary Fiber 2g	8%	Iron	8%
*Percent Daily Values are based on a 2,000 calorie diet			

Strawberry Blueberry Ginger

This spicy and sweet whip is a favorite of those who crave ginger. Add ice if you like a milkshake texture.

2 cups nonfat milk
1 teaspoon flaxseed oil
6 tablespoons protein powder
1 tablespoon wheat germ
1 teaspoon ground ginger
1 cup strawberries
1 cup blueberries

Serves 2

Flaxseeds contain soluble fiber, omega-3 fatty acids, and magnesium, while the wheat germ provides cysteine, an amino acid that plays a major role in removing heavy metals and environmental toxins from our bodies.

SERVING SIZE: ½ OF RECIPE (435G)			
CALORIES: 250		**CALORIES FROM FAT: 35**	
	%DV*		%DV*
Total Fat 4g	6%	Sugars 24g	
Saturated Fat 0.5g	3%	Protein 23g	
Cholesterol 25mg	8%	Vitamin A	10%
Sodium 160mg	7%	Vitamin C	80%
Total Carbohydrate 32g	11%	Calcium	40%
Dietary Fiber 4g	16%	Iron	6%
*Percent Daily Values are based on a 2,000 calorie diet			

Blueberry Banana Smoothie

Try a frozen banana in this creamy delight if you like a thick milkshake texture.

1 cup ice cubes
1 cup milk
1 banana, peeled
½ cup blueberries
½ cup yogurt
1 tablespoon vanilla extract

Serves 1

Yogurt is rich in "good" bacteria that break down toxic bacteria. These friendly flora appear to suppress the growth of bacteria that convert various compounds into carcinogens. Studies show that yogurt helps prevent cancer of the colon and possibly breast cancer. Aim for three to five 8-ounce servings a week.

SERVING SIZE: 1 (799G)			
CALORIES: 400		**CALORIES FROM FAT: 80**	
	%DV*		%DV*
Total Fat 9g	14%	Sugars 43g	
Saturated Fat 4.5g	23%	Protein 17g	
Cholesterol 30mg	10%	Vitamin A	15%
Sodium 220mg	9%	Vitamin C	30%
Total Carbohydrate 60g	20%	Calcium	50%
Dietary Fiber 5g	20%	Iron	4%
*Percent Daily Values are based on a 2,000 calorie diet			

Cherry Freeze

This tart and sweet freeze is better than candy, making it perfect for those with a sweet tooth.

1 cup ice cubes
1 cup fresh cherries, pitted
½ cup cherry juice concentrate
1 tablespoon sweetener

Serves 2

Recent research has identified at least seventeen antioxidant compounds in tart and sweet cherries. A promising group of compounds called anthocyanins has been shown to inhibit enzymes that cause inflammation. Compounds in cherries are currently being researched for their ability to inhibit breast, ovarian, and prostate cancers.

SERVING SIZE: ½ OF RECIPE (279G)			
CALORIES: 280		**CALORIES FROM FAT: 5**	
	%DV*		%DV*
Total Fat 0.5g	1%	Sugars 60g	
Saturated Fat 0g	0%	Protein 3g	
Cholesterol 0mg	0%	Vitamin A	0%
Sodium 95mg	4%	Vitamin C	4%
Total Carbohydrate 67g	22%	Calcium	2%
Dietary Fiber 2g	8%	Iron	8%
*Percent Daily Values are based on a 2,000 calorie diet			

Coffee and Cream

Instant coffee is simply coffee that has been freeze-dried; it reconstitutes easily. The process has been improved over the years, so that newer versions retain their flavorful oils and produce richer cups of coffee.

1 cup milk
½ cup ice cubes
2 tablespoons instant coffee crystals

Serves 1

Coffee is the number-one source of antioxidants in the American diet, says a University of Scranton study. Recently, a group of studies found that drinking coffee daily reduces the potential for liver damage, especially that caused by alcohol consumption: 1 cup a day was found to reduce the chances of liver damage by 20 percent, and 4 cups a day reduced the chances by 80 percent.

SERVING SIZE: 1 (368G)			
CALORIES: 160		**CALORIES FROM FAT: 70**	
	%DV*		%DV*
Total Fat 8g	12%	Sugars 11g	
Saturated Fat 4.5g	23%	Protein 9g	
Cholesterol 25mg	8%	Vitamin A	4%
Sodium 105mg	4%	Vitamin C	0%
Total Carbohydrate 13g	4%	Calcium	30%
Dietary Fiber 0g	0%	Iron	2%
*Percent Daily Values are based on a 2,000 calorie diet			

Pineapple Punch

The sweet pineapple is the predominant flavor in this sparkling punch. This simple combination is perfect for parties or Sunday brunch.

1 frozen peeled banana
½ cup pineapple juice
½ cup orange juice
½ cup sparkling water
1 tablespoon fresh lemon juice

Serves 2

Sparkling water in glass bottles, such as San Faustino, San Pellegrino, and Perrier, is carbonated with CO_2, which is natural and safe. However, other types of carbonation, using phosphoric acid or phosphorus, interfere with mineral absorption and should therefore be avoided. Pineapples contain the enzyme bromelain, and scientists suspect the enzyme interferes with the synthesis of inflammatory substances in the body, such as prostaglandins.

SERVING SIZE: ½ OF RECIPE (250G)			
CALORIES: 110		**CALORIES FROM FAT: 5**	
	%DV*		%DV*
Total Fat 0g	0%	Sugars 20g	
Saturated Fat 0g	0%	Protein 1g	
Cholesterol 0mg	0%	Vitamin A	4%
Sodium 0mg	0%	Vitamin C	70%
Total Carbohydrate 29g	10%	Calcium	2%
Dietary Fiber 2g	8%	Iron	2%
*Percent Daily Values are based on a 2,000 calorie diet			

Peaches and Cream Smoothie

For those who grew up on dairy milk, this may be the perfect introduction to healthy milk alternatives, as the flavor of the soy disappears in this sweet and creamy shake.

1 cup vanilla soymilk
1 cup canned peaches
1 frozen peeled banana
2 tablespoons sweetener
1 teaspoon vanilla extract

Serves 2

Just 1 cup of peaches supplies about 5 percent of the niacin (vitamin B$_3$) we need each day and the carotenoids that the body converts to vitamin A.

SERVING SIZE: ½ OF RECIPE (318G)			
CALORIES: 250		**CALORIES FROM FAT: 15**	
	%DV*		%DV*
Total Fat 2.5g	4%	Sugars 42g	
Saturated Fat 0g	0%	Protein 5g	
Cholesterol 0mg	0%	Vitamin A	10%
Sodium 80mg	3%	Vitamin C	15%
Total Carbohydrate 59g	20%	Calcium	2%
Dietary Fiber 2g	8%	Iron	8%
*Percent Daily Values are based on a 2,000 calorie diet			

Piña Colada Smoothie

This is a classic combination. The tropical flavors really complement each other and bring the taste of the islands right into your kitchen.

1½ cups pineapple nectar
1 cup ice cubes
⅓ cup coconut milk
½ cup pineapple chunks

Serves 2

Components of coconut are currently being studied for their health properties and as an adjunct treatment for bacterial infections such as pneumonovirus, staph, and strep—the most common illnesses brought home from schools every year.

SERVING SIZE: ½ OF RECIPE (389G)			
CALORIES: 200		**CALORIES FROM FAT: 70**	
	%DV*		%DV*
Total Fat 8g	12%	Sugars 30g	
Saturated Fat 7g	35%	Protein 1g	
Cholesterol 0mg	0%	Vitamin A	2%
Sodium 15mg	1%	Vitamin C	25%
Total Carbohydrate 32g	11%	Calcium	4%
Dietary Fiber 1g	4%	Iron	10%
*Percent Daily Values are based on a 2,000 calorie diet			

The Mango Mike

Mike Oros, who lives in Maui and has been making smoothies for years, offered this recipe as his all-time favorite. It is absolutely addictive.

1 cup ice cubes
1 cup mango nectar
1 mango, peeled and pitted
1 banana, fresh or frozen, peeled
Optional: 1 cup vanilla ice cream

Serves 2

Mango is an excellent source of beta-carotene and vitamin C. When you find ripe mangos, buy a case and prepare them for future smoothies. Peel them and slice the flesh away from the pit. Store the mango flesh in a plastic bag in the freezer. Mango nectar, frozen mango slices, mango puree, and mango juice are available in grocery stores and all make great smoothie ingredients.

SERVING SIZE: ½ OF RECIPE (386G)			
CALORIES: 170		**CALORIES FROM FAT: 5**	
	%DV*		%DV*
Total Fat 0g	0%	Sugars 35g	
Saturated Fat 0g	0%	Protein 1g	
Cholesterol 0mg	0%	Vitamin A	30%
Sodium 15mg	1%	Vitamin C	80%
Total Carbohydrate 44g	15%	Calcium	4%
Dietary Fiber 3g	12%	Iron	4%
*Percent Daily Values are based on a 2,000 calorie diet			

Swamp Water Freeze

If you're looking for something less ordinary, try a tea-based smoothie to switch your routine. Tea-based smoothies provide an excellent way to experiment with flavors and intensity, and are perfect when you're looking for something a little less heavy.

2 cups ice cubes
½ cup frozen lemonade concentrate
1 cup frozen tea

Serves 1

Freeze tea ahead of time in ice cube trays to add more flavor. Use any tea you would like, such as chai, black, or herbal tea. You can also make this classic drink with sparkling water. Black tea contains flavanoids, which have been found to lower the risk for vascular problems such as heart attack, stroke, and varicose veins. Tea is a natural source of caffeine, theophylline, and antioxidants.

SERVING SIZE: 1 (856G)				
CALORIES: 260		**CALORIES FROM FAT: 5**		
	%DV*			%DV*
Total Fat 0g	0%	Sugars 60g		
Saturated Fat 0g	0%	Protein 0g		
Cholesterol 0mg	0%	Vitamin A		0%
Sodium 25mg	1%	Vitamin C		45%
Total Carbohydrate 69g	23%	Calcium		2%
Dietary Fiber 1g	4%	Iron		6%
*Percent Daily Values are based on a 2,000 calorie diet				

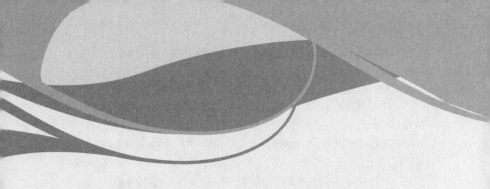

...Alternative
Energy...

In Italy, the little chocolate and espresso-flavored dessert that helps natives get through the late afternoon slump is called *tiramisù*, which literally translates to "pick me up." In England, people have High Tea, and in the United States, our afternoon snack is called "stopping for coffee."

Instead of using a shot of espresso or an energy drink from a can to stimulate the release of adrenaline-like hormones, try something more sustainable. Combine ingredients that give you a lift, but also sustain your energy without depleting and exhausting your adrenal glands.

Energy drinks on the market today contain ingredients that horrify any nutritionist. They include the chemical sweetener sucralose, herbal stimulants such as guarana that are known to cause heart palpitations, blood thinners such as ginkgo biloba, and generally low-quality ingredients such as high-fructose corn syrup, preservatives, and food coloring. The energy is ostensibly supplied by amino acids, B vitamins, and caffeine to stimulate the release of adrenaline. The problem with this strategy is that frequent stimulation of the adrenal glands will eventually drain them, resulting in symptoms such as excessive fatigue, poor memory, headaches, hypoglycemia, dry skin, and even hair loss.

Statistically speaking, many people are routinely turning to energy drinks for their kicks. This is not a sustainable way to meet your energy needs; however it is possible to make smoothies from ingredients that convert stored body fat, blood sugar, and food nutrients into fuel for energy. Not only do we have the food science and nutrition information we need to concoct these energy-producing recipes, we can make them so much tastier at home. By making these smoothies a part of your daily routine, you can infuse your body with nutrients on a regular basis, which increases their medical potency.

Energy Drink Alternatives

You can design your own energy drinks to contain the herbs that are appropriate for your body with the flavors you like and the base liquids your body metabolizes most efficiently.

Most Americans who use medicinal herbs consult with natural health-care physicians, such as oriental medicine doctors, naturopathic physicians, or integrated medicine physicians, to guide them in their choices. Having professional guidance is important in choosing the herbs that are best for meeting your particular needs. The energy drinks sold in grocery stores today contain potent herbs that may or may not be right for you. For example, there are several different types of ginseng, including American, Siberian, and Chinese. Some of these forms stimulate testosterone, which may be fine if you are a fifty-year-old male, but the hormonal effects could be devastating for a woman; testosterone stimulates facial hair growth and imbalances the female hormones. Yikes!

By adding the herbs to your smoothies that your natural health-care practitioner has prescribed for you, you are in essence making personalized medicinal smoothies. This is a wise strategy, as natural medicines like ginseng, guarana, and ephedra may have unwanted effects, such as adrenal depletion, heart palpitations, and even hypoglycemia.

The following recipes are alternatives to the canned and bottled energy drinks sold in today's grocery stores. These recipes have been designed to carry a powerful load of energy-enhancing nutrients that will give you a safe boost if you try them just once, and will have a cumulative effect if you drink them on a regular basis.

Fuel Injection

This light, refreshing drink provides a low-calorie, healthy shot of energy.

1 cup white tea
1 cup sparkling water
1 teaspoon electrolyte powder
1 tablespoon lemon juice
1 tablespoon sweetener
Optional: 1 cup ice cubes

Serves 1

The white tea provides caffeine and antioxidants and the electrolytes support the movement of electrical energy throughout the body. Xylitol is a low-calorie sweetener that helps support the growth of microflora in the digestive tract. One of the health benefits of having healthy colonies of microflora is in their ability to pull B vitamins from the foods you eat. The full range of B vitamins, including folic acid, B_{12}, and B_6, are necessary for energy production.

SERVING SIZE: 1 (514G)					
CALORIES: 70			**CALORIES FROM FAT: 0**		
	%DV*			%DV*	
Total Fat 0g	0%		Sugars 16g		
Saturated Fat 0g	0%		Protein 0g		
Cholesterol 0mg	0%		Vitamin A	0%	
Sodium 0mg	0%		Vitamin C	10%	
Total Carbohydrate 18g	6%		Calcium	15%	
Dietary Fiber 0g	0%		Iron	0%	
*Percent Daily Values are based on a 2,000 calorie diet					

Red Bull Alternative

Get an energy boost from this healthier version of Red Bull, which provides the same benefits without the calories or caffeine.

1 cup sparkling water
1 cup ice cubes
1 capsule taurine powder (the equivalent of 500 mg taurine in powder form)
1 tablespoon sugar
1 teaspoon lime or lemon juice

Serves 1

Taurine is available as a powder and in capsules. Taurine is an amino acid that plays a role in the regulation of body fat metabolism and calcium absorption. It is often added to power drinks for its purported energy-enhancing effects.

SERVING SIZE: 1 (500G)			
CALORIES: 70		**CALORIES FROM FAT: 0**	
	%DV*		%DV*
Total Fat 0g	0%	Sugars 16g	
Saturated Fat 0g	0%	Protein 0g	
Cholesterol 0mg	0%	Vitamin A	0%
Sodium 10mg	0%	Vitamin C	4%
Total Carbohydrate 17g	6%	Calcium	4%
Dietary Fiber 0g	0%	Iron	0%
*Percent Daily Values are based on a 2,000 calorie diet			

Sustained Power

This rich and creamy recipe provides all of the energy-boosting nutrients found in the popular Red Bull product.

1 cup milk
½ cup cottage cheese
3 tablespoons peanut butter
3 tablespoons unsweetened organic cocoa powder
2 tablespoons whey protein powder

Serves 2

This recipe is a powerhouse of nutrients used in various energy-making biochemical pathways. The antioxidants, found in high concentrations in the cocoa, are utilized in energy production. The caffeine from the cocoa dilates blood vessels, increasing circulation of the antioxidants as well as the amino acids.

SERVING SIZE: ½ OF RECIPE (216G)			
CALORIES: 310		**CALORIES FROM FAT: 170**	
	%DV*		%DV*
Total Fat 19g	29%	Sugars 10g	
Saturated Fat 6g	30%	Protein 22g	
Cholesterol 25mg	8%	Vitamin A	6%
Sodium 380mg	16%	Vitamin C	0%
Total Carbohydrate 17g	6%	Calcium	25%
Dietary Fiber 3g	12%	Iron	6%
*Percent Daily Values are based on a 2,000 calorie diet			

Cottage cheese and peanuts are two of the richest vegetarian food sources of methionine known—an amino acid that the liver converts to taurine. In addition, whey protein powder generally contains about 50 mg of taurine-potential per serving.

Taurine is one of the main energy-producing ingredients in drinks such as Red Bull. One theory is that taurine pulls water into the cells, increasing the intracellular metabolism of sugars and increasing energy production as a result. A Japanese study found that rats fed taurine lost weight even on a high-fat diet. This study appears to be the stimulus for the addition of taurine in energy drinks.

Protein Light

This light, frosty drink will take on the flavor of the protein powder you choose. If your protein powder is nonflavored, you may want to add a few drops of vanilla extract.

1 cup rice milk
½ cup ice cubes
3 tablespoons protein powder
1 tablespoon nutritional yeast

Serves 1

The rice-milk base is the least allergenic of the milk bases. Juice can also be used in its place. Protein powder supplies you with all of the amino acids needed for the creation of enzymes, hormones, and neurotransmitters. Water-soluble B vitamins are essential for these same processes and nutritional yeast is packed with them.

SERVING SIZE: 1 (381G)			
CALORIES: 190		**CALORIES FROM FAT: 25**	
	%DV*		%DV*
Total Fat 3g	5%	Sugars 1g	
Saturated Fat 0.5g	3%	Protein 14g	
Cholesterol 25mg	8%	Vitamin A	0%
Sodium 120mg	5%	Vitamin C	2%
Total Carbohydrate 27g	9%	Calcium	15%
Dietary Fiber 1g	4%	Iron	4%
*Percent Daily Values are based on a 2,000 calorie diet			

Port Townsend Mojito

I first tried a Mojito on a boat in the Amazon and fell in love with the fresh mint and lime. To make a smoothie version of this famous drink, first blend the lime with the ice, then add the water and xylitol and blend for a few seconds more. Pour into glasses and garnish with fresh mint leaves. Be sure to add the mint leaves last, as they bruise easily and will become bitter if blended.

2 cups sparkling water
3 cups ice cubes
2 limes, peeled and seeded
2 teaspoons xylitol
4 mint sprigs, leaves only

Serves 4

This recipe contains almost zero calories. The sweetener is xylitol, a low-calorie sugar substitute safe for diabetics, which blends well with citrus and has very little flavor other than a sweet taste. The snap of the limes and hydrating effects of this nonalcoholic drink will perk you up in a heartbeat.

SERVING SIZE: ¼ OF RECIPE (330G)			
CALORIES: 10		**CALORIES FROM FAT: 0**	
	%DV*		%DV*
Total Fat 0g	0%	Sugars 1g	
Saturated Fat 0g	0%	Protein 0g	
Cholesterol 0mg	0%	Vitamin A	0%
Sodium 10mg	0%	Vitamin C	15%
Total Carbohydrate 4g	1%	Calcium	4%
Dietary Fiber 1g	4%	Iron	2%
*Percent Daily Values are based on a 2,000 calorie diet			

ngerade

This refreshing, spicy version of lemonade can be made with lemon or lime. Both are complementary with ginger and sparkling water, and are ultra-refreshing.

1 cup ice cubes
1 teaspoon ground ginger
2 cups sparkling water
1 teaspoon xylitol
½ lemon or lime, peeled

Serves 1

Ginger is an anti-inflammatory and an antioxidant that boosts the immune system and naturally increases the body's energy levels. This drink also counters the damaging effect of dehydration, the most common cause of fatigue.

SERVING SIZE: 1 (741G)			
CALORIES: 15		**CALORIES FROM FAT: 0**	
	%DV*		%DV*
Total Fat 0g	0%	Sugars 1g	
Saturated Fat 0g	0%	Protein 0g	
Cholesterol 0mg	0%	Vitamin A	0%
Sodium 15mg	1%	Vitamin C	25%
Total Carbohydrate 4g	1%	Calcium	8%
Dietary Fiber 1g	4%	Iron	2%
*Percent Daily Values are based on a 2,000 calorie diet			

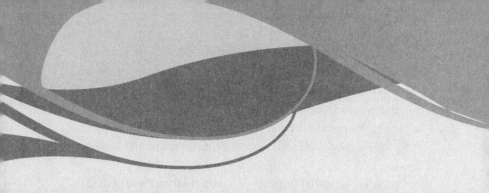

...The Fountain
of Youth...

Slowly but surely, as we age it becomes a little harder to get our systems engaged and moving at the same rate as in our youth. Luckily for us, we are alive in a time of nutritional medicine that has some answers and effective remedies to halt or at least slow down many of the aging processes.

Medical journals regularly reveal new studies on the underlying reasons for the aging of cells and tissues. For example, recent research has found that certain nutritional deficiencies and heavy-metals contamination lead to osteopenia, the main precursor to osteoporosis. We now understand that bone loss is not only caused by a deficiency of calcium, magnesium, and trace minerals but is also precipitated by metals or toxins that block calcium's absorption. We can now halt the progression of this condition by detoxifying the system and replenishing nutrients, and even rebuild porous bones with the right combination of calcium and trace minerals.

Many studies reveal nutrient deficiencies as a root cause of many symptoms of aging. The remedy for deficiencies is to ingest the nutrients you lack, in either food or supplement form.

Supplements work well for vitamin and mineral deficiencies, but are not able to satisfy phytochemical needs, which we are just starting to identify and understand. Phytochemicals are found in produce and have powerful medicinal benefits. By eating the right fruits and vegetables, you can absorb these nutrients, which have a powerful effect on preventing and treating disease.

By adding a regular infusion of a particular nutrient, you can correct a deficiency and often completely reverse the symptoms associated with it. This is good news, as it's becoming more evident that what we have traditionally considered normal aging is often just an imbalance caused by years of poor diet, lack of exercise, and the buildup of toxins. Choosing the right foods gives you the power to prevent and diminish the ravages of time.

Tropical Vista

The variety of exotic fruits in this recipe make for an explosively tasty and interesting beverage.

¼ cup peeled and pitted avocado

1 cup mango juice

1 plum, pitted

1 small peach, peeled and pitted

1 kiwi, peeled

Serves 1

Lutein and zeaxanthin, found in high concentrations in healthy eyes, help shield the eyes from the sun's damaging ultraviolet rays. They also neutralize the free radicals that can damage eyes over time, and those who eat more foods containing lutein and zeaxanthin are less likely to develop age-related macular degeneration (ARMD) or cataracts. Some of the best-known sources of these carotenoids are avocados, plums, peaches, kiwi, and pears. Avocados are also one of the richest studied sources of glutathione, an antioxidant that is part of the glutathione peroxidase enzyme, used by cells to fend off the damage caused by free radicals. In addition, the vitamin E in avocados enhances the anticancer effects of glutathione.

SERVING SIZE: 1 (509G)			
CALORIES: 290		**CALORIES FROM FAT: 60**	
	%DV*		%DV*
Total Fat 6g	9%	Sugars 51g	
Saturated Fat 1g	5%	Protein 3g	
Cholesterol 0mg	0%	Vitamin A	45%
Sodium 15mg	1%	Vitamin C	210%
Total Carbohydrate 62g	21%	Calcium	8%
Dietary Fiber 8g	32%	Iron	10%
*Percent Daily Values are based on a 2,000 calorie diet			

Banana Cocoa Shake

Here the time-tested marriage of cocoa and banana makes for a naturally sweet, dessertlike drink that does much more than satisfy an empty stomach.

1 cup milk
1 frozen peeled banana
¼ cup yogurt
2 tablespoons protein powder
2 tablespoons unsweetened cocoa powder
4 tablespoons ground walnuts

Serves 2

Walnuts contain an omega-3 fatty acid called eicosopentaenoic acid (EPA), which can reduce cataract risk, and the cocoa contains cancer-fighting antioxidants.

SERVING SIZE: ½ OF RECIPE (229G)			
CALORIES: 240		**CALORIES FROM FAT: 100**	
	%DV*		%DV*
Total Fat 11g	17%	Sugars 15g	
Saturated Fat 3g	15%	Protein 13g	
Cholesterol 20mg	7%	Vitamin A	6%
Sodium 90mg	40%	Vitamin C	8%
Total Carbohydrate 26g	9%	Calcium	25%
Dietary Fiber 3g	12%	Iron	6%
*Percent Daily Values are based on a 2,000 calorie diet			

Peanut Swirl

Dates have a sweet subtle flavor, and they combine well with the richness of peanut butter.

1 cup milk
2 dates, pitted and chopped
2 tablespoons peanut butter
2 tablespoons protein powder

Serves 2

Nuts contain vitamin E, which slows the progression of cataract development. Dates are a great source of fiber, potassium, and antioxidants. This is also a delicious way to get a major protein boost.

SERVING SIZE: ½ OF RECIPE (167G)				
CALORIES: 250		**CALORIES FROM FAT: 110**		
	%DV*			%DV*
Total Fat 12g	18%	Sugars 23g		
Saturated Fat 3.5g	18%	Protein 12g		
Cholesterol 20mg	7%	Vitamin A		4%
Sodium 135mg	6%	Vitamin C		0%
Total Carbohydrate 27g	9%	Calcium		20%
Dietary Fiber 3g	12%	Iron		4%
*Percent Daily Values are based on a 2,000 calorie diet				

Radical Neutralizer

This fruity punch is light and refreshing, perfect for a daily afternoon cooler.

1 cup sparkling water
2 tablespoons frozen orange juice concentrate
2 kiwis, peeled
1 cup seedless grapes

Serves 2

Certain carotenoid compounds such as beta cryptoxanthin and zeaxanthin, which are found in kiwi, oranges, and grapes, may help reduce the risk of developing rheumatoid arthritis. They further appear to neutralize the free radicals thought to cause the joint inflammation of rheumatoid arthritis.

SERVING SIZE: ½ OF RECIPE (292G)			
CALORIES: 130		**CALORIES FROM FAT: 5**	
	%DV*		%DV*
Total Fat 0.5g	1%	Sugars 26g	
Saturated Fat 0g	0%	Protein 2g	
Cholesterol 0mg	0%	Vitamin A	4%
Sodium 5mg	0%	Vitamin C	170%
Total Carbohydrate 32g	11%	Calcium	6%
Dietary Fiber 3g	12%	Iron	4%
*Percent Daily Values are based on a 2,000 calorie diet			

Green Fairy

Avocado gives this creamy combination a smooth, rich texture.

1 cup milk
2 tablespoons peanut butter
¼ ripe avocado, peeled and pitted
2 teaspoons nutritional yeast

Serves 1

A new Dutch study found that folic acid may help slow the cognitive decline sometimes associated with aging. Folic acid deficiency was also found to be the cause of many anxiety, stress, and depression disorders. Nutritional yeast contains folic acid as well as all B vitamins.

SERVING SIZE: 1 (328G)			
CALORIES: 420		**CALORIES FROM FAT: 280**	
	%DV*		%DV*
Total Fat 31g	48%	Sugars 14g	
Saturated Fat 8g	40%	Protein 18g	
Cholesterol 25mg	8%	Vitamin A	6%
Sodium 260mg	11%	Vitamin C	8%
Total Carbohydrate 23g	8%	Calcium	30%
Dietary Fiber 6g	24%	Iron	6%
*Percent Daily Values are based on a 2,000 calorie diet			

Painkiller Potion

This medicinal combination can have a profound effect on health, reducing inflammation and pain when taken daily. The orange and lemon juices hide the flavors of many of its blander ingredients.

1 cup milk
1 cup ice cubes
1 cup orange segments
¼ cup frozen lemon juice concentrate

2 tablespoons ground flax-seed
2 tablespoons fish oil supplement
2 tablespoons protein powder

Serves 2

When back- and neck-pain sufferers took a fish oil supplement (1,200 mg daily) for 75 days, 60 percent reported significant pain relief that allowed them to decrease or discontinue use of painkillers. There are many flavored fish-oil supplements available today. Two tubes of Coromega contain the 1,200 mg needed daily to reduce the inflammatory effects at the level of the study; 1,200 mg can also be obtained in 2 tablespoons of most medical-grade flavored fish-oil supplements.

SERVING SIZE: ½ OF RECIPE (410G)			
CALORIES: 320		**CALORIES FROM FAT: 190**	
	%DV*		%DV*
Total Fat 21g	32%	Sugars 17g	
Saturated Fat 5g	25%	Protein 10g	
Cholesterol 95mg	32%	Vitamin A	280%
Sodium 65mg	3%	Vitamin C	110%
Total Carbohydrate 25g	8%	Calcium	25%
Dietary Fiber 7g	28%	Iron	2%
*Percent Daily Values are based on a 2,000 calorie diet			

Macular Miracle

As a daily support for preventing macular degeneration, this combination is powerful medicine—and tasty, too.

1 cup milk
1 frozen peeled banana
½ cup mango nectar
2 tablespoons pumpkin seeds
2 tablespoons almond or macadamia butter
1 tablespoon wheat germ

Serves 2

Grind the pumpkin seeds and nuts first and then add the other ingredients. Those who eat a diet rich in beta-carotene, vitamins C and E, and the mineral zinc can greatly reduce their risk of developing the vision-damaging, age-related macular degeneration (ARMD), which can permanently blur vision over time. Pumpkin seeds are one of the best vegetarian sources of zinc, while nuts contain vitamin E. Choose a beta-carotene-rich fruit for this recipe such as mango, apricot, or cantaloupe.

SERVING SIZE: ½ OF RECIPE (277G)			
CALORIES: 350		**CALORIES FROM FAT: 180**	
	%DV*		%DV*
Total Fat 20g	31%	Sugars 22g	
Saturated Fat 4.5g	23%	Protein 13g	
Cholesterol 10mg	3%	Vitamin A	15%
Sodium 125mg	5%	Vitamin C	25%
Total Carbohydrate 34g	11%	Calcium	20%
Dietary Fiber 4g	16%	Iron	20%
*Percent Daily Values are based on a 2,000 calorie diet			

Strawberry Bone Builder

This strawberry shake is a lovely addition to the nutritional program for those with osteopenia or osteoporosis. It's also a tasty summer drink for anyone with a sweet tooth.

1 cup soymilk
1 cup frozen strawberries

½ cup ice cubes
1 teaspoon vanilla extract

Serves 2

Daily consumption of soymilk, tofu, and other soy-based foods can help protect older women against bone fractures, especially in years immediately following menopause. Strawberries, as well as apples and cucumbers, are excellent sources of vanadium, which is a trace mineral needed for proper calcium absorption.

Participants in a recent large-scale study who were at lowest risk for bone fracture were those who regularly consumed approximately 25 grams of soy food daily—roughly equivalent to 2 cups of soymilk and a large piece of tofu. Soy caveat: If you have thyroid problems or are taking synthroid or other thyroid medication, replace the soy with another milk option, as soy interferes with thyroid hormones.

SERVING SIZE: ½ OF RECIPE (254G)			
CALORIES: 90		**CALORIES FROM FAT: 10**	
	%DV*		%DV*
Total Fat 2.5g	4%	Sugars 5g	
Saturated Fat 0g	0%	Protein 6g	
Cholesterol 0mg	0%	Vitamin A	15%
Sodium 70mg	3%	Vitamin C	50%
Total Carbohydrate 12g	4%	Calcium	6%
Dietary Fiber 3g	13%	Iron	10%
*Percent Daily Values are based on a 2,000 calorie diet			

Power Vision

Frozen bananas are excellent in this nutrient-dense elixir.

1 cup milk
1 cup frozen peeled banana
2 tablespoons whey protein powder
1 tablespoon nutritional yeast
Optional: ½ teaspoon vitamin C powder

Serves 1

Nutritional yeast is a concentrated source of B vitamins. Whey contains glutathione, which helps clean up toxins that have the potential to damage eyesight. The vitamin C protects the eyes from the oxidative damages of the sun, and the fruit provides electrolytes to help the eyes stay hydrated.

SERVING SIZE: 1 (375G)			
CALORIES: 300		**CALORIES FROM FAT: 80**	
	%DV*		%DV*
Total Fat 9g	14%	Sugars 26g	
Saturated Fat 5g	25%	Protein 19g	
Cholesterol 40mg	13%	Vitamin A	6%
Sodium 120mg	5%	Vitamin C	15%
Total Carbohydrate 40g	13%	Calcium	35%
Dietary Fiber 4g	16%	Iron	4%
*Percent Daily Values are based on a 2,000 calorie diet			

Mango Manna

This drink is truly lush and heavenly, especially when you are in the mood for something cold, thick, and sweet to sustain you.

1 cup mango nectar
1 frozen peeled banana
1 cup ice cubes
½ cup yogurt

Serves 1

Carotenoids from the mango offer sun protection, while the banana provides needed potassium, and the yogurt has protein and beneficial microflora. This recipe is great for sun worshippers as it contains nutrients that protect us from ultraviolet rays.

SERVING SIZE: 1 (719G)			
CALORIES: 300		**CALORIES FROM FAT: 5**	
	%DV*		%DV*
Total Fat 0.5g	1%	Sugars 54g	
Saturated Fat 0g	0%	Protein 9g	
Cholesterol 5mg	2%	Vitamin A	45%
Sodium 135mg	6%	Vitamin C	80%
Total Carbohydrate 69g	23%	Calcium	25%
Dietary Fiber 4g	16%	Iron	6%
*Percent Daily Values are based on a 2,000 calorie diet			

Apple Cherry Ginger

This combination is almost like having an apple pie in a glass. Serve it over ice if you like your smoothies very cold. Barley malt is the perfect sweetener for this recipe as it complements the acidic apple-cherry sauce.

2 cups nonfat milk

1 teaspoon flaxseed oil

6 tablespoons protein powder

1 cup apple-cherry sauce

1 teaspoon ground ginger

1 teaspoon barley malt syrup

1 tablespoon wheat germ

Optional: ½ cup ice cubes

Serves 2

Ginger has warming properties and therefore increases circulation to the walls of the digestive tract, which supports digestion and metabolism of food.

Cherry skin is dark red because of its antioxidants called anthocyanins. The antioxidant activity of tart black cherries is greater than that of vitamin E, and so helpful in reducing inflammation and joint pain that it is recommended for those with gout or arthritis.

SERVING SIZE: ½ OF RECIPE (402G)			
CALORIES: 300		**CALORIES FROM FAT: 35**	
	%DV*		%DV*
Total Fat 3.5g	5%	Sugars 16g	
Saturated Fat 0.5g	3%	Protein 23g	
Cholesterol 25mg	8%	Vitamin A	10%
Sodium 200mg	8%	Vitamin C	6%
Total Carbohydrate 44g	15%	Calcium	35%
Dietary Fiber 2g	8%	Iron	6%
*Percent Daily Values are based on a 2,000 calorie diet			

Bones of Steel

This creamy shake is chocolate-almond heaven in a glass.

1 cup fortified milk   2 tablespoons almond butter
½ cup cottage cheese   2 tablespoons whey protein powder
1 cup ice cubes   2 tablespoons cocoa powder

Serves 2

Eating calcium-rich foods is not enough to ensure that the calcium gets absorbed into bones properly. Your body also needs cofactors for the building of bone mass. In this recipe, milk provides calcium and phosphorus, the almond butter has magnesium, and fortified milk contains vitamin D.

> The USDA conducted an experiment in which postmenopausal women took 3 mg of boron per day. The results show that boron can drop unhealthy excretion of calcium by 44 percent. Food sources of this important element include nuts, grains, apples, raisins, and grapes.

SERVING SIZE: ½ OF RECIPE (323G)			
CALORIES: 260		**CALORIES FROM FAT: 150**	
	%DV*		%DV*
Total Fat 16g	25%	Sugars 9g	
Saturated Fat 5g	25%	Protein 18g	
Cholesterol 25mg	8%	Vitamin A	6%
Sodium 330mg	14%	Vitamin C	0%
Total Carbohydrate 14g	5%	Calcium	25%
Dietary Fiber 2g	8%	Iron	6%
*Percent Daily Values are based on a 2,000 calorie diet			

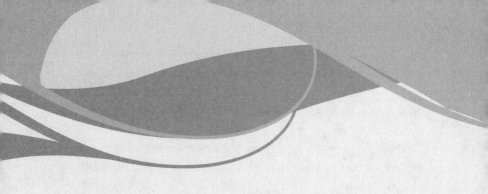

...Beauty from Within...

The influence of nutrition on all aspects of beauty is well known. The attractive attributes we strive for are encompassed by words such as *healthy*, *youthful*, *vibrant*, *lustrous*, *smooth*, and *strong*. Some of the physical signs of beauty are shiny hair, strong nails, youthful skin, white teeth, and a healthy posture that reflects dense bones.

A healthy body pulses with a steady supply of vital nutrients that circulate into our tissues. As our cells are constantly breaking down while new cells are forming, we need the nutrients required to build those cells on hand and ready to work, or those cells will divide without the nutrients they need, resulting in aberrant and fragile growth.

As a clinical nutritionist, I have seen the dramatic effects of nutrient deficiencies and the improvement in appearance after nutrient stores are replaced. One of my patients, a women in her sixties, went gray after an illness. As she replaced her B vitamins, and minerals, her hair color gradually returned.

I have also seen many cases of heavy-metal poisoning from dental amalgams (silver fillings). Unfortunately, when these amalgam fillings are removed, mercury vapors are released and absorbed into the body, where they interfere with bodily processes. An ashen skin color is typical of people suffering from heavy-metal toxicity. The skin color returns when the metals are removed and the minerals are replaced.

Thin, fragile nails are common to people with insufficient protein in their diets. Most of my clients in clinical practice come to me with dry skin from EFA and electrolyte deficiency. After just a few days of replacing these nutrients and drinking plenty of water, their skin becomes as silky as if they had just moisturized with lotion.

A Few Beauty Tips

Graying Hair

Premature graying of the hair is often the result of nutrient deficiencies. It appears that minerals such as zinc, copper, and iron play roles as do water-soluble vitamins such as the B vitamins. Adding them to your diet can reverse these deficiencies, giving your hair the tools it needs to grow properly and allowing the color compounds to reenter the follicles. Choose smoothie ingredients such as copper-rich raisins and almonds, pumpkin seeds and dairy foods for zinc, and citrus for vitamin C. Vitamin C enhances the absorption of many minerals. Nutritional yeast is rich in B vitamins.

Nails

Fingernails and toenails reflect your nutritional status in many ways. Nails are composed of the nutrients that are in your bloodstream at the time they develop. If you have had a deficiency in the past, this will often be seen in the nails as they grow out. The appearance of one's nails may reflect the following deficiencies:

• **Brittle nails** This is often reflective of B vitamin deficiency. The B vitamins are found in nutritional yeast.

- **Spooning nails** This is thought to be a B_{12} deficiency. Adding a tablespoon of nutritional yeast to your diet each day will provide enough B_{12} and the full range of B vitamins to meet your body's needs.
- **White spots** Zinc deficiency often results in white spots on the fingernails. There are several foods that contain zinc that can be added to smoothies to help replace this important mineral. Pumpkin seeds are a good source of zinc.
- **Dry nails** Adding protein to your drinks in the form of nonfat dry milk, cottage cheese, tofu, soy, or nut butter will help support the growth of nails and keep them firm and moist. Most people report that their nails grow faster, they are stronger, and they don't break as easily when they are getting sufficient protein. Essential fatty acids (EFAs) help reduce inflammation that may occur around the nails. EFAs are found in fish oil, flaxseed oil, and borage seed oil.
- **Peeling nails** If your nails begin peeling, this may be a sign that you need more vitamin A. Adding carotenoids to your diet will help your body to convert them into vitamin A as needed. Taking vitamin A as a supplement can be risky, as your body does not have a way to flush out the excess vitamin A. It can build up to toxic levels that supress the immune system.
- **Ridges** These may be reflective of a malabsorption of nutrients. Taking supplemental digestive enzymes can help improve your body's absorption.

Skin

- **Dry skin** When our skin is dry, it is a warning sign that we may be dehydrated. To stay well hydrated, take in ample amounts of water, electrolytes, and EFAs every day. Add sparkling water and ice to your smoothies to increase the water content. Fruits and vegetables contain electrolyte minerals, or you can take specific electrolyte supplements, which are available in powder or liquid form. Ground flaxseed, flaxseed oil, and flavored fish oils are all great EFA sources for smoothies.

- **Acne** Bioflavonoids and zinc help kill the bacteria that cause acne. Pumpkin seeds and animal products such as milk and cottage cheese are sources of zinc. Bioflavonoids such as hesperetin, hesperidin, eriodictyol, quercetin, and rutin are found in the white material just beneath the peel of citrus fruits and in black currants.
- **Wrinkles** Support the production of collagen by adding vitamin C from citrus fruits and carotenoids from orange fruits to your recipes.

Bones and Teeth

Calcium, and the minerals that support its absorption, will help your bones and teeth stay strong. Vitamins D, B_6, B_{12}, and folic acid, as well as the elements magnesium, boron, and vanadium, are required for proper absorption of calcium. Vanadium food sources are oats, cooked rice, and wheat germ. Boron food sources include apples, grapes, nuts, and grains. The B vitamins (including B_6 and B_{12}) can be obtained from nutritional yeast. Vitamin D food is found in sunflower seeds and wheat germ.

Smoothie Ingredients for Beauty Enhancement

Vitamin C

Vitamin C from foods such as citrus fruit and strawberries or supplements is important for manufacturing the protein collagen, the building material for connective tissue, cartilage, and tendons. Aim for 2 to 3 grams per day.

Carotenoids

Carotenoids are antioxidants that protect the skin from the sun's damaging rays and protect the eyes from many oxidation-related diseases. Mixed carotenoids from apricots, peaches, cherries, papayas, persimmons, citrus fruits, pumpkin, cantaloupe, and watermelon will all help protect the skin from environmental damage.

Copper

The mineral copper is needed only in tiny quantities in our diets. It is found in wheat, prunes, nuts, and cocoa, which are all perfect smoothie ingredients. Copper is one of the constituents in hair color.

Digestive Enzymes

Often a bloated abdomen is caused by maldigestion. Take digestive enzymes with your smoothie or add enzyme powder directly to your smoothie for a flatter stomach every day.

Essential Fatty Acids

Essential fatty acids (EFAs) such as docosahexaenoic acid (DHA) and eicosapentaenoic acid (EPA) are found in fish oil. Gamma-linolenic acid (GLA) is found in plants such as primrose, borage, and flaxseed. These fats are needed to help keep us hydrated, to make our skin smooth, and to reduce inflammation. For those who are deficient, taking EFAs provides almost immediate relief from dry skin, brittle nails, puffy tissues, and dehydrated, wrinkled skin.

Glutathione

Glutathione is a sulfur-containing nutrient that helps remove environmental toxins and heavy metals from our tissues. When contaminated with metal from fish, dental amalgams, or other metal sources, skin can become ashen and gray. When the metals are removed, the elasticity returns along with a youthful glow.

Microflora

The organisms in our digestive tract known as microflora play a major role in the metabolism of B vitamins. Medications such as antibiotics damage our microflora. One way to replace them is by taking capsules or powdered microflora supplements. These organisms help keep the digestive tract clean and healthy, and they reduce the toxic burden on the body, which translates directly to cleaner tissues and less frequent infection. Yogurt is an excellent food source of microflora and probiotics.

Protein

Protein-rich foods such as dairy, nuts, and soyfoods contain amino acids that the body uses to make skin, hair, nails, and blood cells. Your body needs a constant supply of these amino acids as it is in a continual process of breaking down old tissue and replacing it.

Sulfur

Sulfur is present in every cell in the body. It is a necessary building block for the growth of hair, skin, and nails. Sulfur is a main component in vitamins such as thiamine, pantothenic acid, and biotin. Dairy foods, eggs, onions, and garlic all contain sulfur.

Zinc

Zinc is a very important mineral found in pumpkin seeds and animal products such as dairy foods. Zinc supports the immune system, assists in muscle regeneration, helps our bodies repair damaged tissue, helps our immune systems clean up bacteria within the body, and is necessary for healthy eyes.

Power Nails

If taken daily, this creamy shake can make a difference in nail texture within just a few weeks. A luxurious white beverage, it goes down surprisingly smooth.

1 cup milk
½ cup cottage cheese
1 cup ice cubes
1 teaspoon flaxseed oil
1 teaspoon vanilla extract
Optional: 2 tablespoons unsweetened cocoa powder
        1 tablespoon liquid calcium

Serves 1

The calcium and protein available in this dense concoction do wonders to strengthen dry and brittle nails, as they are key components in their growth and production.

SERVING SIZE: 1 (604G)			
CALORIES: 300		**CALORIES FROM FAT: 150**	
	%DV*		%DV*
Total Fat 17g	26%	Sugars 16g	
Saturated Fat 8g	40%	Protein 21g	
Cholesterol 40mg	13%	Vitamin A	10%
Sodium 510mg	21%	Vitamin C	0%
Total Carbohydrate 16g	5%	Calcium	40%
Dietary Fiber 0g	0%	Iron	0%
*Percent Daily Values are based on a 2,000 calorie diet			

Pink Passion

When you're in the mood for something fruity but fast, just think pink!

4 cups seedless watermelon

Serves 1

My beautiful Danish friend, Janneke, introduced me to "just watermelon." It's full of skin-protecting carotenoids, which neutralize the oxidizing effects of the environment.

> Drink this alone without food and then wait 30 minutes before eating, as most people digest melon better on an empty stomach.

SERVING SIZE: 1 (608G)			
CALORIES: 180		**CALORIES FROM FAT: 10**	
	%DV*		%DV*
Total Fat 1g	2%	Sugars 38g	
Saturated Fat 0g	0%	Protein 4g	
Cholesterol 0mg	0%	Vitamin A	70%
Sodium 5mg	0%	Vitamin C	80%
Total Carbohydrate 46g	15%	Calcium	4%
Dietary Fiber 2g	8%	Iron	8%
*Percent Daily Values are based on a 2,000 calorie diet			

Skin Glow

The raisins and hazelnuts in this yummy recipe make for a spicy, snappy taste sensation.

½ cup almond milk
½ cup yogurt
¼ cup raisins
¼ cup sliced almonds or hazelnuts
1 tablespoon toasted wheat germ
1 tablespoon flaxseed oil

Serves 2

Essential fatty acids in flax oil help hydrate the skin, while the magnesium in the nuts helps to circulate nutrients through the skin's small capillaries in the skin. The raisins offer iron to carry oxygen to the cells. Think of this drink as your daily "internal" facial.

SERVING SIZE: ½ OF RECIPE (168G)			
CALORIES: 280		**CALORIES FROM FAT: 130**	
	%DV*		%DV*
Total Fat 14g	32%	Sugars 24g	
Saturated Fat 1g	5%	Protein 8g	
Cholesterol 0mg	0%	Vitamin A	8%
Sodium 100mg	4%	Vitamin C	2%
Total Carbohydrate 33g	11%	Calcium	20%
Dietary Fiber 3g	12%	Iron	8%
*Percent Daily Values are based on a 2,000 calorie diet			

Youth Elixir

Adding frozen, rather than fresh, berries gives this formula a thick milkshake texture.

½ cup milk
½ cup vanilla yogurt
½ cup frozen blackberries
1 tablespoon nutritional yeast

Serves 1

The focus in this recipe is the glutathione in the milk and yogurt, the antioxidants in the berries, and the probiotics contained in yogurt. The B vitamins in the nutritional yeast support healthy skin development.

SERVING SIZE: 1 (314G)			
CALORIES: 200		**CALORIES FROM FAT: 50**	
	%DV*		%DV*
Total Fat 6g	9%	Sugars 21g	
Saturated Fat 3.5g	18%	Protein 11g	
Cholesterol 20mg	7%	Vitamin A	8%
Sodium 130mg	5%	Vitamin C	6%
Total Carbohydrate 26g	9%	Calcium	35%
Dietary Fiber 5g	20%	Iron	4%
*Percent Daily Values are based on a 2,000 calorie diet			

Rose Petal

This drink is a glowing tribute to the underappreciated flavor of strawberries, which partner perfectly with bananas and other mild fruits.

1 cup strawberry juice
1 cup ice cubes
1 tablespoon flaxseed oil
1 frozen peeled banana
1 teaspoon electrolyte powder

Serves 2

Give your skin youthful softness with essential fatty acids such as those found in flaxseed oil. Electrolytes help the skin hydrate, filling in fine lines and giving the skin a plump, youthful look.

SERVING SIZE: ½ OF RECIPE (305G)			
CALORIES: 150		**CALORIES FROM FAT: 70**	
	%DV*		%DV*
Total Fat 7g	11%	Sugars 15g	
Saturated Fat 0.5g	3%	Protein 1g	
Cholesterol 0mg	0%	Vitamin A	2%
Sodium 5mg	0%	Vitamin C	60%
Total Carbohydrate 22g	7%	Calcium	8%
Dietary Fiber 2g	8%	Iron	4%
*Percent Daily Values are based on a 2,000 calorie diet			

Chocolate Banana Shake

Cottage cheese is such a wonderful addition to smoothies because it becomes so creamy. The decadent taste and lush texture of this shake make it a perfect substitute for a standard dessert.

1 cup ice cubes
½ cup milk
1 cup cottage cheese
1 frozen peeled banana
1 tablespoon unsweetened cocoa powder
2 tablespoons sweetener

Serves 2

If you use an organic cocoa powder such as Dagoba, you will be adding antioxidants, which protect the skin from the oxidative stress that ages cells. High-protein foods such as cottage cheese contain amino acids that the body uses to build strong nails, healthy skin, and thick, luxuriant hair.

SERVING SIZE: ½ OF RECIPE (376G)			
CALORIES: 260		**CALORIES FROM FAT: 60**	
	%DV*		%DV*
Total Fat 7g	11%	Sugars 30g	
Saturated Fat 4g	20%	Protein 16g	
Cholesterol 20mg	7%	Vitamin A	8%
Sodium 430mg	18%	Vitamin C	8%
Total Carbohydrate 39g	13%	Calcium	20%
Dietary Fiber 2g	8%	Iron	2%
*Percent Daily Values are based on a 2,000 calorie diet			

Fruit Fresh

The bright flavors of this frozen fruit blend are highlighted by the fresh lemon juice.

¼ cup frozen grapes
½ frozen peeled banana
½ cup milk
1 teaspoon lemon juice
2 tablespoons cottage cheese

Serves 1

Grapes contain flavonoids such as resveratrol that protect the skin from environmental damage, and the banana provides potassium, a key electrolyte in hydrating tissue. Well-hydrated skin is younger looking and less prone to flaking and breakouts.

SERVING SIZE: 1 (314G)			
CALORIES: 230		**CALORIES FROM FAT: 50**	
	%DV*		%DV*
Total Fat 6g	9%	Sugars 27g	
Saturated Fat 3g	15%	Protein 9g	
Cholesterol 15mg	5%	Vitamin A	6%
Sodium 150mg	6%	Vitamin C	30%
Total Carbohydrate 41g	14%	Calcium	15%
Dietary Fiber 3g	12%	Iron	2%
*Percent Daily Values are based on a 2,000 calorie diet			

Teen Scene

This orange, creamy whip is tasty enough to drink every day and perfect for teenagers as breakfast or an afternoon snack.

1 cup orange juice
1 cup ice cubes
1 small orange, peeled with a knife (see Note)
¼ cup nonfat dry milk powder
¼ cup pumpkin seeds

Serves 2

This drink is helpful in clearing acne and preventing bacterial infections, owing to the protective effects of the bioflavonoids provided by the oranges and the zinc from the pumpkin seeds.

NOTE: Use a knife to cut away just the orange outside skin, while leaving the white pithy part of the skin intact. The white parts of the skin contain the bioflavonoids.

SERVING SIZE: ½ OF RECIPE (326G)			
CALORIES: 250		**CALORIES FROM FAT: 110**	
	%DV*		%DV*
Total Fat 12g	18%	Sugars 20g	
Saturated Fat 2g	10%	Protein 13g	
Cholesterol 0mg	0%	Vitamin A	15%
Sodium 60mg	3%	Vitamin C	150%
Total Carbohydrate 27g	9%	Calcium	15%
Dietary Fiber 2g	8%	Iron	25%
*Percent Daily Values are based on a 2,000 calorie diet			

Mango Madness

Combining fresh mango with mango nectar gives this smoothie a divine fresh-off-the-island flavor.

1 cup ice cubes
1 cup mango nectar
1 fresh mango, peeled and pitted
1 banana, fresh or frozen, peeled

Serves 2

Mango contains concentrated carotenoids that support healthy, youthful skin. If you drink this one daily for a few weeks, your skin will start to take on the color of the carotenoids, giving you a beautiful, fresh glow.

SERVING SIZE: ½ OF RECIPE (386G)			
CALORIES: 170		**CALORIES FROM FAT: 5**	
	%DV*		%DV*
Total Fat 0g	0%	Sugars 35g	
Saturated Fat 0g	0%	Protein 1g	
Cholesterol 0mg	0%	Vitamin A	30%
Sodium 15mg	1%	Vitamin C	80%
Total Carbohydrate 44g	15%	Calcium	4%
Dietary Fiber 3g	12%	Iron	4%
*Percent Daily Values are based on a 2,000 calorie diet			

GMP

The classic Hawaiian combination of guava, mango, and papaya is reminiscent of lazy days at the beach.

1 cup ice cubes
½ cup guava nectar
½ cup mango nectar
½ papaya, peeled and seeded
Optional: ½ cup yogurt

Serves 2

One serving of papaya will meet about 20 percent of an adult's daily folate needs, and it provides about 75 percent of an adult's daily vitamin C needs. Both folate and vitamin C are integral nutrients in creating collagen. By providing the body with the nutrients needed to build new collagen, you can reduce the development of wrinkles.

SERVING SIZE: ½ OF RECIPE (279G)			
CALORIES: 80		**CALORIES FROM FAT: 0**	
	%DV*		%DV*
Total Fat 0g	0%	Sugars 18g	
Saturated Fat 0g	0%	Protein 0g	
Cholesterol 0mg	0%	Vitamin A	15%
Sodium 15mg	1%	Vitamin C	70%
Total Carbohydrate 21g	7%	Calcium	2%
Dietary Fiber 1g	4%	Iron	2%
*Percent Daily Values are based on a 2,000 calorie diet			

Pumpkin Glow

This whip is light yet filling. The fresh pumpkin seeds and blueberries make for a surprising but yummy combination.

¼ cup pumpkin seeds
1 cup milk
½ cup blueberries
¼ cup toasted wheat germ
¼ teaspoon microflora or 1 tablespoon yogurt
2 tablespoons protein powder

Serves 2

The pumpkin seeds provide zinc, which boosts the immune system and helps clear bacteria from the body, including the infections involved in acne breakouts. The blueberries are rich in antioxidants, which reduce oxidation (aging) of skin; the wheat germ provides vitamin E, the fat-soluble antioxidant.

TIP: Grind the nuts in a dry blender or food processor first, then add wet ingredients.

SERVING SIZE: ½ OF RECIPE (214G)			
CALORIES: 330		**CALORIES FROM FAT: 160**	
	%DV*		%DV*
Total Fat 18g	28%	Sugars 13g	
Saturated Fat 4.5g	13%	Protein 22g	
Cholesterol 20mg	7%	Vitamin A	6%
Sodium 70mg	3%	Vitamin C	6%
Total Carbohydrate 22g	7%	Calcium	20%
Dietary Fiber 5g	20%	Iron	30%
*Percent Daily Values are based on a 2,000 calorie diet			

Cranberry Protection

Whipping frozen berries with juice results in a bright, simple drink that is clean and fresh on the palate.

1 cup ice cubes
1 cup cranberry juice
1 cup frozen berries
1 teaspoon sweetener

Serves 2

Cranberries are rich in vitamin C, a powerful antioxidant that protects cells from damage from environmental toxins and stress.

SERVING SIZE: ½ OF RECIPE (324G)			
CALORIES: 120		**CALORIES FROM FAT: 5**	
	%DV*		%DV*
Total Fat 0g	0%	Sugars 26g	
Saturated Fat 0g	0%	Protein 1g	
Cholesterol 0mg	0%	Vitamin A	2%
Sodium 10mg	0%	Vitamin C	25%
Total Carbohydrate 30g	10%	Calcium	4%
Dietary Fiber 4g	16%	Iron	6%
*Percent Daily Values are based on a 2,000 calorie diet			

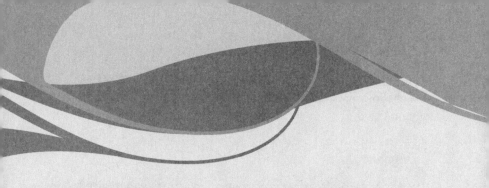

...Fat Burners...

The biochemistry of body-fat storage is fascinating and complex. Most of my clients are specifically interested in weight loss, and together we try to work out a regimen based on individual habits and needs. However, there are some basic, common imbalances that lead to increased body-fat storage and low metabolism no matter what your body type, meaning that there are many strategies that are effective.

By supporting hormone pathways, neurotransmitter signals, and the metabolic pathways directly responsible for triggering the use of stored fat as energy, we can directly increase our metabolism and burn more body fat. Proper hydration, improved thyroid function, an increased intake of dietary protein, and a nutrient-rich diet are all important to this process. Nutrients such as coenzyme Q_{10} (commonly called CoQ10), minerals, and essential fatty acids also support the metabolic systems, and a deficiency in any of them can cause metabolism and enzymatic pathways to work at an extremely slow pace. By replacing these deficiencies with the important metabolic elements, you can start the pathways functioning normally again, which makes a dramatic difference in terms of fat loss.

General Guidelines

The following approaches are helpful not only in supporting weight loss and body-fat elimination but also for improving general health.

Hydrate

Dehydration results in reduced metabolic activity and reduced fat-burning ability. On a daily basis, most of us are so dehydrated that our metabolic function has slowed down as a result. Medical studies from the University of Washington have found that by rehydrating our bodies we instantly restore our metabolic function by between 3 and 5 percent, depending on the level of dehydration, which changes by the hour. Drinking water, taking in electrolytes via food supplements, and getting the essential fatty acids we need from fish and plants will restore hydration almost immediately. To minimize exposure to plastic bottles, use filtered tap water or European bottled water such as Pellegrino, Perrier (with or without gas), or San Faustino calcium water, which are bottled in glass.

Improve Thyroid Function and Absorption

Low thyroid function is a common cause of slow metabolism and can be improved by eating iodine-rich foods such as milk, cottage cheese, and yogurt. Avoid soy foods if you have low thyroid function as the phytochemicals in soybeans block the absorption of thyroid.

Choose Protein Foods

Taking in enough daily protein helps to stabilize blood sugar and reduce sugar cravings, resulting in less calorie intake and less insulin production (as both encourage fat storage).

Plant proteins contain soluble and insoluble fiber that help hydrate and cleanse the intestine, allow healthy microflora to prosper, give the feeling of satiety, and maintain blood sugar levels. Take in approximately 100 grams of protein (see protein chart) from plant sources daily.

> ● ● ●
>
> Participants in a Johns Hopkins study noted that they felt more full and had less appetite when they ate more protein. Researchers at the University of Washington School of Medicine in Seattle tested two diets—15 percent protein for two weeks, then 30 percent protein for two weeks. The higher protein diet group lost an average of 11 pounds more over twelve weeks.

Increase Your Antioxidants

Antioxidants from concentrated sources such as green tea, blueberries, pomegranate, chocolate, and vegetables reduce oxidation in the cells. Antioxidants work with CoQ10 to enhance the enzymatic action in fat cells, which allows stored fat to release into the bloodstream and be used for energy.

Look for B Vitamins

Vitamin B_1 (thiamine), vitamin B_2 (riboflavin), vitamin B_3 (niacin), vitamin B_5 (pantothenic acid), vitamin B_6 (pyridoxine and pyridoxamine), folicin (folic acid), and vitamin B_{12} (cyanocobalamin) are the B vitamins. They work synergistically, meaning they work better when taken together. The B vitamins increase oxygen transportation, which improves energy production and cleaner burning of fuel. These nutrients can be obtained from supplements or foods such as nutritional yeast. Be wary of foods such as coffee, sugar, white flour, and alcohol, which deplete the B vitamins in your bloodstream and increase your need for B vitamins.

Eat Healthy Fats to Control Cravings

Unhealthy fats aren't needed or used by the body the same way essential fatty acids (EFAs) are. Unhealthy fats, when eaten in excess, end up stored in fat cells, whereas EFAs are absorbed and used in skin, joint tissue, and biochemical pathways that help reduce inflammation.

A diet rich in EFAs reduces fat cravings. Avoid hydrogenated fats, trans fats, and saturated fats, which offer little nutritional value and have a heavy caloric load. A diet low in these unhealthy fats improves blood flow so that blood can physically move through the vessels, carrying oxygen and nutrients to improve muscle action and enzymatic action in the fat cells.

Increase your consumption of plant fats from nuts, seeds, and avocados to meet gamma-linolenic acid (GLA) requirements and small fish, or flavored fish oil supplements, to meet Eicosapentaenoic acid (EPA) and docosahexaenoic acid (DHA) needs. These essential fats also reduce inflammation (thus reducing water retention), balance prostaglandins (reducing menstrual cramps and colon spasms), and are absorbed by the skin and tissues, so there is no danger that these fats will end up stored in fat cells.

Don't Starve Yourself

Starvation slows the burning of body fat by reducing enzymatic activity in the cells. Eat generous amounts of whole foods from sources such as beans, peas, lentils, fish, vegetables, whole grains, and whole fruit. Eating a whole-foods diet rather than restricting your calories will improve your metabolism.

Drink Breakfast

Eating breakfast every day is an important factor for keeping off weight. A bowl of steel-cut oats and a piece of fruit, or a smoothie with protein powder or cottage cheese added to it, starts your day with stable blood sugar. Brown University Medical School researchers found that 78 percent of their study participants who achieved lasting weight loss ate breakfast daily. An earlier study from the University of Massachusetts found that people who habitually missed the morning meal were four times more likely to be obese.

Reduce Inflammation

Visceral fat is more metabolically active than other types of fat and produces a chemical reaction that triggers inflammation. As you start to lose weight, you will lose visceral fat, which then reduces inflammation. This cycle enhances the burning of body fat.

Inflammation is a response of the immune system to infection or irritation, which is outwardly seen as redness, heat, swelling, and pain and can result in dysfunction of the organs. Internal inflammation wreaks havoc on many systems. The degree of inflammation in the body can be monitored by a simple blood test that measures C-reactive protein, a powerful inflammatory marker. Studies have found it to be effective in predicting the risk of conditions such as heart disease and the presence of food allergies.

• • •

A 2005 study from the Harvard School of Public Health found that women who ate high-fiber diets rich in fruits, vegetables, and whole grains had lower levels of C-reactive protein than women whose diets consisted primarily of refined grains.

• • •

A 2004 study in the journal *Psychosomatic Medicine* found that anger and depression both elevated the levels of C-reactive protein in otherwise healthy people.

Food allergies can cause dramatic inflammation around the digestive tract. For many, this results in abdominal water weight gain that can be as high as 15 pounds. When food allergies are treated, the immune system stops reacting and the water is released through the urinary system, resulting in many pounds of weight loss, especially for those with immunoglobin G (IgG) food allergies.

Nutrients That Increase Fat Burning

Replacing lost nutrients that are known to affect metabolism and body-fat burning can help correct biochemical malfunctions.

Minerals

Improve muscle action, glycogen burning, and energy production with calcium and magnesium-containing foods. These foods include nuts, seeds, nut butters, and dairy products. Both liquid calcium and powdered magnesium blend well in smoothies.

Trace Minerals

Trace minerals such as chromium improve glucose transportation into the cells, which stops sugar cravings immediately. Nuts and seeds contain chromium and can be added to smoothies in the form of nut butters.

Coenzyme Q_{10}

Coenzyme Q_{10} (CoQ10) deficiency results in a reduced ability to produce the enzymes needed to break down body fat. Increasing CoQ10 via supplements or whole foods can restore enzymatic action in fat cells, allowing the release of stored fat. Toasted wheat germ is the perfect CoQ10-containing food to add to smoothies as it blends well, has very little taste, and almost disappears in a creamy drink.

Fiber

Add whole fruits that are fresh, frozen, or dried and fiber products such as psyllium seed powder or ground flaxseed.

Water

Add water to smoothies in the form of purified tap water, bottled carbonated water, or ice cubes.

Protein

Protein food sources for smoothies include dairy foods such as cottage cheese, nonfat dry milk powder, milk, and yogurt, as well as plant foods such as tofu, nuts, seeds, and nut butter.

Quercetin

Quercetin, a flavonoid, directly inhibits several initial processes of inflammation, resulting in water weight loss. Apples, citrus fruits, berries, green tea, and cocoa contain quercetin.

Taurine

A deficiency in taurine leads to reduced fat metabolism. Our bodies make taurine from methionine. Food sources of methionine include cottage cheese and peanuts. We must also take in B_6 for our livers to make the conversion from methionine to taurine.

Green Tea

Green tea contains four main catechin substances: catechin (EC), epicatechin gallate (ECG), epigallocatechin (EGC), and epigallocatechin gallate (EGCG). These antioxidants reduce body-fat storage and are believed to be one of the main reasons women in Asia have less body fat than women in other countries.

Berries

Cyanidin is a natural organic compound found in berries, classified as both a flavonoid and an anthocyanin. It provides the pigment for many red berries including, but not limited to, bilberries, blackberries, blueberries, cherries, cranberries, elderberries, hawthorns, loganberries, and raspberries. It can also be found in other fruits such as apples and plums.

Green Tea Ice Cream

If you've never tried green tea ice cream, now's your chance! This frosty drink is just as good as the dessert—and healthier, too.

1 cup milk
1 cup ice cubes
½ cup green tea
¼ cup açaí juice
2 tablespoons wheat germ
1 tablespoon sweetener

Serves 2

Green tea contains bioflavonoids, polyphenols, and powerful antioxidants. These catechins support the production of enzymes in the fat cells to break down body fat and release it into the bloodstream, where it can be burned as you exercise.

SERVING SIZE: ½ OF RECIPE (348G)			
CALORIES: 150		**CALORIES FROM FAT: 40**	
	%DV*		%DV*
Total Fat 4.5g	7%	Sugars 18g	
Saturated Fat 2.5g	13%	Protein 6g	
Cholesterol 10mg	3%	Vitamin A	2%
Sodium 55mg	2%	Vitamin C	0%
Total Carbohydrate 21g	7%	Calcium	15%
Dietary Fiber 2g	8%	Iron	4%
*Percent Daily Values are based on a 2,000 calorie diet			

Cherry Apple Cooler

Fruit juice concentrates are loaded with nutrients and taste. Just a few tablespoons of concentrate have the flavor of 1 cup of juice, but are as rich as liquors without the alcohol. Eden, the makers of organic juices, also make fruit juice concentrates and many of them are organic.

1 cup ice cubes
1 cup sparkling water
2 tablespoons cherry concentrate
2 tablespoons frozen apple juice concentrate

Serves 1

Japanese studies suggest that cyanidin, found in concentration in cherries, may aid in preventing obesity and diabetes and may reduce inflammation.

SERVING SIZE: 1 (549G)			
CALORIES: 160		**CALORIES FROM FAT: 0**	
	%DV*		%DV*
Total Fat 0g	0%	Sugars 35g	
Saturated Fat 0g	0%	Protein 1g	
Cholesterol 0mg	0%	Vitamin A	0%
Sodium 65mg	3%	Vitamin C	50%
Total Carbohydrate 38g	13%	Calcium	6%
Dietary Fiber 0g	0%	Iron	6%
*Percent Daily Values are based on a 2,000 calorie diet			

Green Tea Frosty

This Margarita-like slushee is light and refreshing, especially after exercise, and can be a daily part of a weight-loss program.

1 cup green tea
1 cup ice cubes
1 tablespoon lemon juice
1 tablespoon sweetener

Serves 1

Researchers at the University of Geneva, Switzerland, found that green tea has thermogenic properties and promotes fat burning.

SERVING SIZE: 1 (510G)			
CALORIES: 70		**CALORIES FROM FAT: 0**	
	%DV*		%DV*
Total Fat 0g	0%	Sugars 16g	
Saturated Fat 0g	0%	Protein 0g	
Cholesterol 0mg	0%	Vitamin A	0%
Sodium 10mg	0%	Vitamin C	10%
Total Carbohydrate 18g	6%	Calcium	0%
Dietary Fiber 0g	0%	Iron	0%
*Percent Daily Values are based on a 2,000 calorie diet			

Pomegranate Power Icy

The tart citrus flavor of this light icy is a refreshing cocktail at any hour.

1 cup pomegranate juice
½ cup lemonade concentrate
½ cup ice cubes
1 tablespoon wheat germ

Serves 2

Coenzyme Q_{10} works in conjunction with antioxidants to help stimulate the release of stored body fat. One tasty source of CoQ10 is wheat germ, which blends well in smoothies. Green tea, blueberries, and pomegranate are all highly touted antioxidant sources. Use a combination of these juices if you have them on hand, as a blend of antioxidants has been found to be more effective than a single antioxidant alone.

SERVING SIZE: ½ OF RECIPE (262G)			
CALORIES: 220		**CALORIES FROM FAT: 5**	
	%DV*		%DV*
Total Fat 0.5g	1%	Sugars 48g	
Saturated Fat 0g	0%	Protein 2g	
Cholesterol 0mg	0%	Vitamin A	0%
Sodium 20mg	1%	Vitamin C	20%
Total Carbohydrate 54g	18%	Calcium	2%
Dietary Fiber 1g	4%	Iron	6%
*Percent Daily Values are based on a 2,000 calorie diet			

Apple Frosty

Simple and sweet! This combination is so easy and delicious that it may become a daily favorite.

1 cup apple juice
1 frozen peeled banana

Serves 1

One of the reasons the amount of body fat we carry seems to change dramatically from day to day is that fat contains a tremendous amount of water. When we reduce inflammation, we support our body's ability to let go of this water. Apples contain quercetin, which is effective in reducing the inflammation that causes water retention.

SERVING SIZE: 1 (366G)			
CALORIES: 220		**CALORIES FROM FAT: 5**	
	%DV*		%DV*
Total Fat 0g	0%	Sugars 41g	
Saturated Fat 0g	0%	Protein 1g	
Cholesterol 0mg	0%	Vitamin A	2%
Sodium 0mg	0%	Vitamin C	25%
Total Carbohydrate 56g	9%	Calcium	0%
Dietary Fiber 3g	12%	Iron	4%
*Percent Daily Values are based on a 2,000 calorie diet			

Strawberry Protein Shake

So creamy and sweet, yet so good for weight loss. Plus it's filling enough to satisfy your cravings between meals.

1 cup milk
1 cup frozen strawberries
½ cup cottage cheese

Serves 1

Cottage cheese contains protein and methionine, which the liver converts to taurine, the amino acid known for increasing fat metabolism. Also, strawberries contain fiber, which slows their digestion, thus helping to regulate blood sugar and minimize the release of the fat-storage hormone insulin.

SERVING SIZE: 1 (507G)			
CALORIES: 300		**CALORIES FROM FAT: 110**	
	%DV*		%DV*
Total Fat 13g	20%	Sugars 22g	
Saturated Fat 8g	40%	Protein 21g	
Cholesterol 40mg	13%	Vitamin A	10%
Sodium 500mg	21%	Vitamin C	100%
Total Carbohydrate 29g	10%	Calcium	40%
Dietary Fiber 3g	12%	Iron	6%
*Percent Daily Values are based on a 2,000 calorie diet			

Protein Power

Choose a low-calorie sweetener, such as those made from herbs like stevia, a chicory-based product like Just Like Sugar, or a sugar alcohol such as xylitol.

1 cup milk
½ cup cottage cheese
¼ cup unsweetened cocoa powder
2 tablespoons toasted wheat germ
1 tablespoon nutritional yeast
1 tablespoon sweetener

Serves 2

This combination really packs a punch to body fat. The protein in the milk and cheese helps stabilize blood sugar levels, thus reducing the production of insulin, the fat-storage hormone. The antioxidants in the cocoa support the actions of CoQ10, provided in this recipe by the toasted wheat germ. (CoQ10 helps the enzymes in the fat cells break down body fat and release it from fat cells.) Also, the nutritional yeast supplies the B vitamins necessary for metabolic function.

SERVING SIZE: 1 (209G)			
CALORIES: 220		**CALORIES FROM FAT: 70**	
	%DV*		%DV*
Total Fat 8g	12%	Sugars 17g	
Saturated Fat 4g	20%	Protein 15g	
Cholesterol 20mg	7%	Vitamin A	6%
Sodium 250mg	10%	Vitamin C	0%
Total Carbohydrate 26g	9%	Calcium	20%
Dietary Fiber 4g	16%	Iron	8%
*Percent Daily Values are based on a 2,000 calorie diet			

a Freeze

This is a refreshing alternative to iced tea and oh-so-much healthier for you.

1 cup apple juice
1 cup tea, preferably green or white tea
2 cups ice cubes
Optional: ½ teaspoon vitamin C powder

Serves 2

A recent study found that green tea, which contains both tea catechins and caffeine, inhibits enzymes called catechol O-methyl-transferase and phosphodiesterase to battle obesity. Apple juice serves as a natural sweetener that satisfies sugar cravings without a lot of calories.

SERVING SIZE: ½ OF RECIPE (479G)			
CALORIES: 60		**CALORIES FROM FAT: 0**	
	%DV*		%DV*
Total Fat 0g	0%	Sugars 14g	
Saturated Fat 0g	0%	Protein 0g	
Cholesterol 0mg	0%	Vitamin A	0%
Sodium 10mg	0%	Vitamin C	2%
Total Carbohydrate 15g	5%	Calcium	0%
Dietary Fiber 0g	0%	Iron	2%
*Percent Daily Values are based on a 2,000 calorie diet			

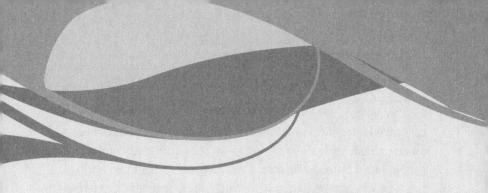

...Brain Boosters...

The *Journal of Nutritional Health and Aging* reported that an increase in oxidative stress, from factors such as poor diet or exposure to environmental toxins, contributes to a decline in cognitive performance. There are many promising studies that define the role of phytochemicals in the prevention and treatment of neurological conditions such as memory loss as well as Alzheimer's and Parkinson's diseases.

It is clear that inflammation, too, plays a role in many cognitive problems. The *Annals of Neurology* reported that the fewest cases of neurological diseases were seen in people who ate a Mediterranean diet rich in fruits, vegetables, legumes, fresh fish, and olive oil. A nutrient known for its ability to help reduce inflammation, lecithin, is a special type of fat called a phospholipid; its chemical name is phosphatidylcholine. It contains choline, which is a promising nutrient for improving memory. Lecithin can be found in wheat germ and peanut butter.

Together, these medical studies guide us to eat more fresh fruits and vegetables that are rich in phytochemicals, essential fatty acids that reduce inflammation, and nutrients that help detoxify our systems.

General Nutrition Guidelines

Apples

Researchers at Cornell University found that a group of chemicals called phenolics, which are naturally occurring antioxidants found in fresh apples, can protect nerve cells from the neurotoxicity induced by oxidative stress and can protect the brain from the type of damage that triggers such neurodegenerative diseases as Alzheimer's and Parkinson's. Apple juice, fresh apple slices, liquid apple juice concentrate, frozen apple juice concentrate, and applesauce are all good choices for smoothies.

Blueberries

Recent studies of blueberries found that there can be cognitive improvements from the consumption of such polyphenolic-rich fruits. The components of the blueberry thought to be responsible for this miraculous effect are their powerful antioxidants and phytochemicals, such as anthocyanins, ellagic acid, catechins, and resveratrol.

Cherries

Cherry anthocyanins have been shown to reduce pain and inflammation.

Choline

When choline was fed to pregnant rats, their offspring showed significantly better memory in maze tests than rats whose mothers were not fed choline. And the improved memory was maintained at a level comparable to that of much younger rats even after the rats grew old. The beneficial effect probably relates to lecithin's function in nerve membranes and to the need for choline to make the neurotransmitter acetylcholine, which enables signals to go from nerve to nerve. Lecithin granules and liquid are made from soybeans.

Coenzyme Q$_{10}$

Coenzyme Q$_{10}$ has long been used to treat high blood pressure, heart disease, cancer, and Parkinson's disease. In a recent study, migraine sufferers who took 100 milligrams of liquid CoQ10 three times a day for three months averaged only 3.2 migraines per month versus 4.4 migraines per month before the study. Those who received a placebo reported no change. CoQ10 is found in wheat germ.

Green Tea

The catechins in green tea have been found repeatedly in tests to improve cognitive function in adults. Catechins are antioxidants that scavenge and remove the debris that is thought to cause many degenerative cognitive diseases.

Ginger

Ginger has a long history of medicinal use as an anti-inflammatory agent for a wide variety of diseases, pain, and neurodegenerative conditions such as Alzheimer's and Parkinson's diseases. Inflammatory diseases, including cancer, atherosclerosis, myocardial infarction, diabetes, allergies, asthma, arthritis, Crohn's disease, multiple sclerosis, osteoporosis, psoriasis, septic shock, and AIDS, respond when inflammation is reduced through the use of ginger extracts. Ginger extract also inhibits the expression of a wide range of inflammation-related genes.

Walnuts

Walnuts contain essential fatty acids that support the development of brain cells and neurotransmitters.

Tropical Frosty

This is a delightful smoothie to make for a friend. It's light and refreshing, made from a universally loved combination of fruits, plus it helps protect a most valuable asset—the brain.

1 cup sparkling water
1 cup ice cubes
½ cup pineapple juice
¼ cup mango juice or puree
¼ cup coconut juice
2 tablespoons lecithin

Serves 2

Lecithin is a phospholipid that is attracting the attention of researchers because it may reduce age-related memory loss. It is nontoxic, inexpensive, and extremely good for cell membranes and the skin. Coconut juice is a good source of electrolytes to help move the electrical impulses of the body through the brain, and vitamin C (from the fruit) protects brain cells from oxidative degeneration.

SERVING SIZE: ½ OF RECIPE (367G)			
CALORIES: 160		**CALORIES FROM FAT: 90**	
	%DV*		%DV*
Total Fat 10g	15%	Sugars 12g	
Saturated Fat 6g	30%	Protein 1g	
Cholesterol 0mg	0%	Vitamin A	4%
Sodium 10 mg	0%	Vitamin C	15%
Total Carbohydrate 14g	5%	Calcium	6%
Dietary Fiber 0g	0%	Iron	8%
*Percent Daily Values are based on a 2,000 calorie diet			

Peanut Butter Shake

Peanut butter and cottage cheese may not sound like natural partners, but when combined, these two always make for thick, opulent drinks full of flavor and nutrients.

1 cup milk

1 cup ice cubes

1 tablespoon nutritional yeast

1 tablespoon peanut butter

1 teaspoon lecithin granules

¼ cup cottage cheese

Serves 1

Cottage cheese provides methionine, a nutrient used in the manufacture of taurine, which both provides amino acids for cardiac function and serves in the brain and gut as a neurotransmitter. The lecithin contains choline, which the body uses to create an important sheath over the nerves to protect them as they carry messages throughout the body. Nutritional yeast supplies the B vitamins needed for nerve cell production, and peanut butter provides the amino acids that are the building blocks for nerves, brain cells, and other neurotransmitters.

SERVING SIZE: 1 (560G)			
CALORIES: 320		**CALORIES FROM FAT: 180**	
	%DV*		%DV*
Total Fat 20g	31%	Sugars 14g	
Saturated Fat 8g	40%	Protein 20g	
Cholesterol 30mg	10%	Vitamin A	8%
Sodium 380mg	16%	Vitamin C	0%
Total Carbohydrate 18g	6%	Calcium	35%
Dietary Fiber 2g	8%	Iron	4%
*Percent Daily Values are based on a 2,000 calorie diet			

Raspberry Whip

This apple-berry combination is creamy and slightly sweet with just a hint of tartness from the juice. Just delicious!

1 cup raspberries
1 cup apple juice
¼ cup cottage cheese
Optional: ¼ teaspoon vitamin C powder

Serves 2

Raspberries contain anthocyanins and ellagic acid. The anthocyanins in berries protect brain cells from age-related decline. An exciting new study demonstrated that apple juice concentrate prevents an increase in oxidative damage to brain tissue that can lead to a decline in cognitive performance.

SERVING SIZE: ½ OF RECIPE (214G)			
CALORIES: 110		**CALORIES FROM FAT: 15**	
	%DV*		%DV*
Total Fat 1.5g	2%	Sugars 17g	
Saturated Fat 1g	5%	Protein 4g	
Cholesterol 5mg	2%	Vitamin A	2%
Sodium 100mg	4%	Vitamin C	30%
Total Carbohydrate 23g	8%	Calcium	4%
Dietary Fiber 4g	16%	Iron	4%
*Percent Daily Values are based on a 2,000 calorie diet			

Orange Banana Cream

This creamy orange shake is so scrumptious you may want to drink it every day. This is a great way to get sustained release benefits of the nutrients in smoothies!

1 cup orange juice
1 fresh or frozen peeled banana
3 tablespoons protein powder
1 tablespoon flaxseed oil
1 tablespoon nutritional yeast
1 tablespoon toasted wheat germ

Serves 1

This is a great drink to have the morning of a test or a presentation. The protein powder provides amino acids, the flaxseed contains the essential fatty acids needed for calming and focusing, the nutritional yeast is packed with B vitamins (which are cofactors in many neurological processes), and the banana offers potassium for the electrical current to carry messages through the body and brain. The wheat germ provides CoQ10, which helps prevent migraines.

SERVING SIZE: 1 (405G)			
CALORIES: 440		**CALORIES FROM FAT: 140**	
	%DV*		%DV*
Total Fat 16g	25%	Sugars 37g	
Saturated Fat 2g	10%	Protein 19g	
Cholesterol 25mg	8%	Vitamin A	10%
Sodium 35mg	1%	Vitamin C	220%
Total Carbohydrate 58g	19%	Calcium	15%
Dietary Fiber 6g	24%	Iron	10%
*Percent Daily Values are based on a 2,000 calorie diet			

Cherry, Ginger, Peach

EdenBlend Rice & Soy Beverage is the perfect base for this rich and creamy smoothie, and the cherry juice concentrate gives it great flavor.

2 cups Rice & Soy Beverage
1 teaspoon flaxseed oil
6 tablespoons protein powder
1½ tablespoons tart cherry juice concentrate
1 teaspoon barley malt syrup or honey
1 teaspoon ground ginger
2 cups frozen sliced peaches

Serves 4

A recent study suggests that ginger extract may be useful in delaying the onset and progression of neurodegenerative disorders. These disorders are often attributed to some degree of brain inflammation, which is also thought to contribute to the neuron loss associated with Alzheimer's disease.

SERVING SIZE: ¼ OF RECIPE (209G)			
CALORIES: 160		**CALORIES FROM FAT: 25**	
	%DV*		%DV*
Total Fat 3g	5%	Sugars 16g	
Saturated Fat 0.5g	3%	Protein 10g	
Cholesterol 10mg	3%	Vitamin A	4%
Sodium 70mg	12%	Vitamin C	120%
Total Carbohydrate 22g	7%	Calcium	8%
Dietary Fiber 1g	4%	Iron	6%
*Percent Daily Values are based on a 2,000 calorie diet			

Peanut Cream Whip

By making this sweet treat a daily part of your health routine, you are literally feeding your brain the amino acids it needs to stay sharp.

1 cup milk
½ cup cottage cheese
¼ cup creamy peanut butter

Serves 2

Methionine is an essential amino acid that plays a role in cognitive function and neurological activity. Cottage cheese and peanuts are both excellent source of methionine.

SERVING SIZE: ½ OF RECIPE (211G)			
CALORIES: 310		**CALORIES FROM FAT: 200**	
	%DV*		%DV*
Total Fat 22g	34%	Sugars 10g	
Saturated Fat 6g	30%	Protein 18g	
Cholesterol 20mg	7%	Vitamin A	6%
Sodium 400mg	17%	Vitamin C	0%
Total Carbohydrate 14g	5%	Calcium	20%
Dietary Fiber 3g	12%	Iron	4%
*Percent Daily Values are based on a 2,000 calorie diet			

rappé

There have never been more health reasons to drink coffee than now. This is yet another delicious excuse. By making coffee drinks at home, you can choose organic ingredients and use healthful sweeteners. Coffee tends to be a daily routine for those who partake in this age-old ritual, so it's important that your drink is high quality. For example, use organic instant coffee as organic coffee products have the highest antioxidant levels.

1 cup milk

1 cup ice cubes

2 teaspoons instant
  coffee crystals

1 teaspoon sweetener

½ teaspoon vanilla extract

2 teaspoons nonfat dry
  milk powder

Serves 2

A recent study found that drinking 24 ounces of coffee a day decreases the risk of Parkinson's disease by about 40 percent and the risk for Alzheimer's disease by about 20 percent. Use xylitol as your sweetener as it helps promote healthy gut flora and improves digestion, and be sure to add the nonfat dry milk to supply a little protein to help get you started in the morning.

SERVING SIZE: ½ OF RECIPE (247G)			
CALORIES: 90		**CALORIES FROM FAT: 35**	
	%DV*		%DV*
Total Fat 4g	6%	Sugars 9g	
Saturated Fat 2.5g	13%	Protein 5g	
Cholesterol 10mg	3%	Vitamin A	4%
Sodium 60mg	3%	Vitamin C	0%
Total Carbohydrate 10g	3%	Calcium	15%
Dietary Fiber 0g	0%	Iron	0%
*Percent Daily Values are based on a 2,000 calorie diet			

Cold Chaud Chocolate

Use a dark chocolate and organic cocoa powder for the most health benefits and richest flavor.

1 cup milk
1 cup ice cubes
3 tablespoons unsweetened cocoa powder
2 tablespoons lecithin
2 tablespoons sweetener

Serves 2

The theobromine content in cocoa stimulates the brain as it is a xanithine similar to coffee, while chocolate is a potent source of antioxidants that help prevent degenerative diseases. Even the lecithin in this recipe help protect brain cells from aging.

SERVING SIZE: ½ OF RECIPE (277G)			
CALORIES: 220		**CALORIES FROM FAT: 80**	
	%DV*		%DV*
Total Fat 9g	14%	Sugars 22g	
Saturated Fat 3.5g	18%	Protein 5g	
Cholesterol 10mg	3%	Vitamin A	2%
Sodium 55mg	2%	Vitamin C	0%
Total Carbohydrate 28g	9%	Calcium	15%
Dietary Fiber 1g	4%	Iron	6%
*Percent Daily Values are based on a 2,000 calorie diet			

Banana Shake

Frozen bananas create a wonderful texture in smoothies, similar to milkshakes. I'd recommend this simple, healthful treat to anyone.

1 cup milk
2 frozen peeled bananas
2 tablespoons lecithin
Optional: ¼ teaspoon ground cinnamon

Serves 2

A study from the University of Camerino in Italy (September 2006) found that the memories of participants who took just 2 tablespoons of lecithin daily for five weeks improved significantly. The investigators concluded that "the cost of lecithin is so low, the negative side effects so minimal, and the potential benefits so positive, that we would recommend all persons experiencing memory problems to take lecithin granules as food supplements." Lecithin is also available in liquid form, which is perfect for smoothies.

SERVING SIZE: ½ OF RECIPE (248G)			
CALORIES: 240		**CALORIES FROM FAT: 80**	
	%DV*		%DV*
Total Fat 8g	12%	Sugars 20g	
Saturated Fat 3.5g	18%	Protein 5g	
Cholesterol 10mg	3%	Vitamin A	4%
Sodium 50mg	2%	Vitamin C	15%
Total Carbohydrate 33g	11%	Calcium	15%
Dietary Fiber 3g	12%	Iron	4%
*Percent Daily Values are based on a 2,000 calorie diet			

Green Tea Frosty

The studies on green tea's health benefits just keep rolling in, and this is one of the easiest and tastiest ways to take advantage of them.

1 cup green tea
1 cup ice cubes
1 cup milk
1 teaspoon sweetener

Serves 2

A 2006 study showed that elderly Japanese people who drank more than 2 cups of green tea a day had a 50 percent lower chance of developing cognitive impairment than those who drank less green tea or who consumed other tested beverages.

SERVING SIZE: ½ OF RECIPE (362G)			
CALORIES: 80		**CALORIES FROM FAT: 35**	
	%DV*		%DV*
Total Fat 4g	6%	Sugars 8g	
Saturated Fat 2.5g	13%	Protein 4g	
Cholesterol 10mg	3%	Vitamin A	2%
Sodium 55mg	2%	Vitamin C	0%
Total Carbohydrate 8g	3%	Calcium	15%
Dietary Fiber 0g	0%	Iron	0%
*Percent Daily Values are based on a 2,000 calorie diet			

...Detoxifiers...

When we have less toxic load in our bodies, our health improves dramatically; most of us have more energy, get sick less, and generally look a whole lot better. Reducing the intake of toxins is, of course, the first step in any detoxification process. Our livers, white blood cells, and enzymatic pathways generally do a great job of breaking down substances that do harm and moving them out of the body through our sweat glands and the digestive and urinary tracts. But a large portion of the population has a genetic predisposition for reduced ability to produce the enzymes that cleave toxins. For these people especially, it is important to avoid toxic substances from the start.

Toxins are all around you, but you can reduce our exposure to them in several ways. You can reduce the intake of chlorine, heavy metals, and organisms such as giardia by filtering your water at the tap. Solid-carbon, activated-charcoal filters, and reverse-osmosis systems are all efficient ways of doing this. Home air filters similarly clean the air we breathe. Choosing whole foods and organic foods rather than packaged, over-processed goods can dramatically reduce the amount of agricultural chemicals, hormones, antibiotics, and other toxic compounds you take in, as can using less toxic shampoos, perfumes, deodorants, and cleaning supplies. Recent studies by the Environmental Working Group (www.EWG.org) have concluded that we are exposed to far more toxins inside the house than outside. I take comfort in knowing that we have more control than we may have thought over our exposure to environmental toxins.

Once you reduce your exposure, the next step is to clean up the toxins in your body. Many detoxification pathways move the toxins from fat cells into the bloodstream and then out through the urinary tract and the digestive tract. But chronic constipation stops the whole process and creates toxemia in the colon. Cancer-causing chemicals from the environment are reabsorbed rather than expelled. To correct this imbalance, take in healthful probiotics from supplements or yogurt and get plenty of insoluble and soluble fiber, which are found in fruits such as plums and prunes. Drink at least 64 ounces of pure water every day and get regular exercise.

Strategies for Detoxification

Reduce Toxic Load

Many toxic substances are eliminated from the system via the digestive tract. As such, daily bowel movements are critical to a clean colon. If you become constipated, try increasing your consumption of water, fiber, and essential fatty acids in order to flush out the toxins and encourage elimination.

Increase Dietary Fiber

Dietary fiber acts like a toxin sponge, absorbing waste materials from the digestive tract and moving them out through the bowels.

Choose Organic Foods

Food produced according to organic standards are grown without the use of chemical pesticides and herbicides, antibiotics, or hormones. Furthermore, the land that organic foods are grown on is free of sewage sludge. When you buy foods labeled "organic," you can also rest assured that they have not been genetically engineered. This is important when detoxing, because genetically engineered plant foods have a higher level of chemical residue and lower nutritional value than their organic counterparts.

Increase Your Water Consumption

Water assists many biochemical actions that clear toxins and infections in the body. Add mineral water, ice, or sparkling water to smoothies to increase water content.

Include Electrolytes

Liquid or powdered electrolytes help the body absorb water.

Look for Essential Fatty Acids

Essential fatty acids (EFAs) help cells stay hydrated once they absorb water. Add flaxseed oil or flavored fish oils to your smoothies to increase their EFA content.

Follow a Whole Foods Diet

A whole-foods diet is based on foods that are minimally processed, without added food coloring, preservatives, or flavorings. Whole foods for smoothies include fruits, vegetables, grains (e.g., rolled oats, cooked brown rice, or cooked quinoa), nuts, and seeds.

Avoid Toxins

Try to avoid exposure to toxins such as chlorine by purifying your tap water, to chemicals by purchasing organic foods, to environmental chemicals by decreasing or rethinking your use of lawn-care products, and to toxic personal care and cleaning products (shampoos, perfumes, and deodorants) by opting for natural brands.

Increase the Detoxifying Nutrients

Probiotics or microflora colonize in the digestive tract and help remove toxins as well as support healthy digestion. These can be added to smoothies from capsules, via yogurt, or in powdered form.

Glutathione, a natural component of whey, is very effective in removing specific toxins such as heavy metals from the body. It can be found in dairy products such as milk, yogurt, nonfat dry milk, cottage cheese, and cream.

Banana Yogurt Frosty

This sweet and creamy blend is a gentle detoxifier.

1 cup ice cubes
½ apple juice
½ cup yogurt
1 frozen peeled banana
¼ cup pitted prunes
1 tablespoon toasted wheat germ
1 teaspoon ground flaxseed

Serves 2

Oats and wheat germ are sources of the powerful free-radical scavenger cysteine. Free radicals form when we are exposed to everyday toxins such as chlorine in our water or pesticide residue on our foods.

SERVING SIZE: ½ OF RECIPE (310G)			
CALORIES: 150		**CALORIES FROM FAT: 5**	
	%DV*		%DV*
Total Fat 1g	2%	Sugars 22g	
Saturated Fat 0g	0%	Protein 6g	
Cholesterol 0mg	0%	Vitamin A	8%
Sodium 65mg	3%	Vitamin C	10%
Total Carbohydrate 33g	11%	Calcium	10%
Dietary Fiber 3g	12%	Iron	4%
*Percent Daily Values are based on a 2,000 calorie diet			

Lemongrass Lemonade

This light, refreshing slushy has a subtle, sweet flavor from the watermelon and the agave nectar. Agave syrup is the sap of a cactus plant. Lemongrass contains oils that have been used in aromatherapy to help relieve nervous tension and stress, giving this smoothie a calming effect. Watermelon is a great detoxifier, as it is full of water and electrolytes.

1 cup lemongrass tea, chilled
1 cup seedless watermelon
   pulp

2 cups ice cubes
¼ cup lemon juice
1 tablespoon agave nectar

Serves 2

Steep the lemongrass tea bag in 8 ounces of hot water for about 2 minutes, then chill the tea before adding it to the smoothie. If you are preparing smoothies for a group of people or just want to have more tea on hand, fill a glass pitcher with hot water and steep several tea bags for 5 minutes, then remove the bags and refrigerate the pitcher. Tea keeps well when refrigerated for about five days.

SERVING SIZE: ½ OF RECIPE (472G)			
CALORIES: 60		**CALORIES FROM FAT: 0**	
	%DV*		%DV*
Total Fat 0g	0%	Sugars 13g	
Saturated Fat 0g	0%	Protein 1g	
Cholesterol 0mg	0%	Vitamin A	8%
Sodium 10mg	0%	Vitamin C	35%
Total Carbohydrate 16g	5%	Calcium	2%
Dietary Fiber 0g	0%	Iron	2%
*Percent Daily Values are based on a 2,000 calorie diet			

Apple Flax Slushy

This simple mix tastes both wholesome and crisp. Here the flaxseed and whey complement the tartness of the apples and make for a pleasant drinking experience.

½ cup apple juice
2 tablespoons ground flaxseed
1 cup ice cubes
1 apple, peeled, seeded, and sliced
1 tablespoon whey protein powder

Serves 1

Flaxseed provides the essential fatty acids that help reduce inflammation and flush our bodies of toxins.

> The predominant phenolic phytochemicals in apples are quercetin, epicatechins, and procyanidin. These are powerful antioxidants that relieve symptoms of environmental allergies.

SERVING SIZE: 1 (492G)			
CALORIES: 190		**CALORIES FROM FAT: 20**	
	%DV*		%DV*
Total Fat 2.5g	4%	Sugars 25g	
Saturated Fat 0g	0%	Protein 8g	
Cholesterol 10mg	3%	Vitamin A	0%
Sodium 20mg	1%	Vitamin C	10%
Total Carbohydrate 37g	12%	Calcium	6%
Dietary Fiber 7g	28%	Iron	2%
*Percent Daily Values are based on a 2,000 calorie diet			

Hi-C

This sweet frosty is like a childhood cherry punch. Add ice and it becomes a nutrient-packed slurpee.

10 fresh cherries, pitted
1 cup sparkling water
1 teaspoon vitamin C powder
1 teaspoon sweetener
Optional: 1 cup ice cubes

Serves 1

Cherries contain concentrated amounts of the powerful free-radical-scavenging anthocyanins. They also are excellent sources of the antioxidant vitamin C, which neutralizes many toxins in the body.

SERVING SIZE: 1 (454G)			
CALORIES: 160		**CALORIES FROM FAT: 15**	
	%DV*		%DV*
Total Fat 1.5g	2%	Sugars 29g	
Saturated Fat 0g	0%	Protein 2g	
Cholesterol 0mg	0%	Vitamin A	0%
Sodium 0mg	0%	Vitamin C	10%
Total Carbohydrate 40g	13%	Calcium	6%
Dietary Fiber 5g	20%	Iron	0%
*Percent Daily Values are based on a 2,000 calorie diet			

Cherrific Apple

This creamy combination of sweet cherries and apple juice is a popular smoothie for those who want to pack in the nutrients without the calories.

10 fresh cherries, pitted
1 cup apple juice
½ cup yogurt
1 cup ice cubes

Serves 1

Dairy foods contain whey, which is a good source of glutathione. Glutathione is an important metals detoxifier, as it binds with heavy metals and helps remove them from the body.

SERVING SIZE: 1 (808G)			
CALORIES: 310		**CALORIES FROM FAT: 15**	
	%DV*		%DV*
Total Fat 15g	2%	Sugars 60g	
Saturated Fat 0g	0%	Protein 9g	
Cholesterol 5mg	2%	Vitamin A	10%
Sodium 125mg	5%	Vitamin C	20%
Total Carbohydrate 73g	24%	Calcium	25%
Dietary Fiber 5g	20%	Iron	2%
*Percent Daily Values are based on a 2,000 calorie diet			

Cinnamon Apple Detoxifier

Sweet with a hint of warm spice, this blend is the perfect accompaniment to a bowl of cereal or oatmeal.

½ cup applesauce
½ cup prune juice
2 tablespoons wheat germ
½ teaspoon ground cinnamon
Optional: ½ pear, cored and seeded
          1 cup ice cubes

Serves 1

Prunes and prune juice are good sources of naturally occurring sorbitol, a natural laxative, as are pears and apples. This is a great drink to add to the daily routine to help move toxins out of your system.

SERVING SIZE: 1 (272G)			
CALORIES: 250		**CALORIES FROM FAT: 15**	
	%DV*		%DV*
Total Fat 2g	3%	Sugars 24g	
Saturated Fat 0g	0%	Protein 5g	
Cholesterol 0mg	0%	Vitamin A	0%
Sodium 45mg	2%	Vitamin C	15%
Total Carbohydrate 56g	19%	Calcium	4%
Dietary Fiber 6g	24%	Iron	20%
*Percent Daily Values are based on a 2,000 calorie diet			

Lemon Meringue

Fresh lemon juice is the key to this perfect whip. It's tart and creamy, with a fresh citrus scent.

½ cup cottage cheese
½ cup milk
½ frozen peeled banana
2 tablespoons lemon juice

Serves 1

The milk, cottage cheese, and whey protein provide glutathione, a detoxifier that binds to heavy metals and other environmental toxins to remove them from the body, thus improving mineral absorption and antioxidant levels in the blood.

SERVING SIZE: 1 (326G)			
CALORIES: 230		**CALORIES FROM FAT: 80**	
	%DV*		%DV*
Total Fat 9g	14%	Sugars 17g	
Saturated Fat 5g	25%	Protein 18g	
Cholesterol 25mg	8%	Vitamin A	10%
Sodium 450mg	19%	Vitamin C	30%
Total Carbohydrate 26g	9%	Calcium	25%
Dietary Fiber 2g	8%	Iron	2%
*Percent Daily Values are based on a 2,000 calorie diet			

Berry Lime Blast

Rich, bright, and absolutely loaded with detoxifying phyto-chemicals.

½ cup cranberry juice
½ cup frozen raspberries
½ cup blueberries
1 teaspoon honey
1 teaspoon lime juice

Serves 1

Eating a variety of brightly colored fruit each day is important because the colors in the plant foods are physical evidence of the actual nutrients, such as the red anthocyanin of grapes. A broad diet rich in such phytonutrients will yield thousands of different polyphenol antioxidants, which assist in detoxifying various chemical compounds.

SERVING SIZE: 1 (326G)			
CALORIES: 170		**CALORIES FROM FAT: 5**	
	%DV*		%DV*
Total Fat 0g	0%	Sugars 34g	
Saturated Fat 0g	0%	Protein 2g	
Cholesterol 0mg	0%	Vitamin A	4%
Sodium 0mg	0%	Vitamin C	70%
Total Carbohydrate 43g	14%	Calcium	2%
Dietary Fiber 3g	12%	Iron	6%
*Percent Daily Values are based on a 2,000 calorie diet			

ueberry Lemon Sorbet

This bright purple delight is sweet with just a hint of lemon.

1 cup frozen blueberries
½ cup orange juice
1 teaspoon honey
1 teaspoon lemon juice

Serves 1

Recent tests on the antioxidant effectiveness of various fruits put blueberries and oranges at the top of the list. They are most effective against the damaging oxidative processes that take place in the cells.

SERVING SIZE: 1 (291G)			
CALORIES: 160		**CALORIES FROM FAT: 10**	
	%DV*		%DV*
Total Fat 1g	2%	Sugars 29g	
Saturated Fat 0g	0%	Protein 2g	
Cholesterol 0mg	0%	Vitamin A	6%
Sodium 0mg	0%	Vitamin C	110%
Total Carbohydrate 38g	13%	Calcium	2%
Dietary Fiber 4g	16%	Iron	2%
*Percent Daily Values are based on a 2,000 calorie diet			

Apple Lime

Fresh, cold, and sweet with just a hint of citrus, this simple drink is delicious.

1 cup applesauce
1 cup ice cubes
½ teaspoon lime juice

Serves 1

Applesauce contains powerful detoxifying agents, such as the antioxidants polyphenols and glutathione.

SERVING SIZE: 1 (495G)				
CALORIES: 190		**CALORIES FROM FAT: 5**		
	%DV*			%DV*
Total Fat 0g	0%	Sugars 0g		
Saturated Fat 0g	0%	Protein 0g		
Cholesterol 0mg	0%	Vitamin A		0%
Sodium 80mg	3%	Vitamin C		8%
Total Carbohydrate 51g	17%	Calcium		2%
Dietary Fiber 3g	12%	Iron		4%
*Percent Daily Values are based on a 2,000 calorie diet				

Plum Freeze

This sparkling fruity drink is a healthy start to each day, and a great way to incorporate plums into your diet.

1 cup pitted plums
1 cup sparkling water
1 cup ice cubes
Optional: 1 teaspoon xylitol

Serves 2

Plums are also a natural source of sorbitol, a sugar alcohol that acts as a laxative.

SERVING SIZE: ½ OF RECIPE (350G)			
CALORIES: 50		**CALORIES FROM FAT: 5**	
	%DV*		%DV*
Total Fat 0g	0%	Sugars 11g	
Saturated Fat 0g	0%	Protein 1g	
Cholesterol 0mg	0%	Vitamin A	8%
Sodium 5mg	0%	Vitamin C	20%
Total Carbohydrate 13g	4%	Calcium	2%
Dietary Fiber 2g	8%	Iron	2%
*Percent Daily Values are based on a 2,000 calorie diet			

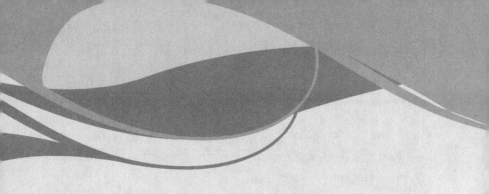

...Immune
Boosters...

Chronic illness, bacterial infections, fungal infections such as *Candida* overgrowth, poor wound healing, fatigue syndromes, and cancer are all signs of a suppressed immune system. We count on our white blood cells to protect us from invaders, but their production and activity are largely dependent on our diets. Our immune system is severely compromised when we are deficient in one or more of the nutrients needed for white blood cells to work. We further suppress our immune function when we eat sugar, do not get enough protein, and do not give our bodies the antioxidants they need to clean up unhealthy free radicals.

Strategies for Supporting the Immune System

By reducing our sugar intake, increasing our dietary protein, and eating foods that contain antioxidants, we can improve immune function to a great degree.

Reduce Sugar Use

Reduce sugar intake, which suppresses white blood cell production. Avoid refined sugars, sweeteners, and white flour products, which break down into sugar quickly. The same goes for refined breads, pastries, and sweetened products. To sweeten smoothies, use natural, low-sugar sweeteners such as Just Like Sugar, xylitol, and stevia.

Increase Protein Intake

Protein foods such as cottage cheese, nonfat dry milk, yogurt, nuts, seeds, nut butters, and protein powder contain amino acids that strengthen cell walls and help ward off disease.

Avoid Nutrient Deficiencies

The following list summarizes how specific nutrient deficiencies affect the immune system.

- **Zinc** A shortage in zinc causes a decrease in T cells and natural killer (NK) cell activity.
- **Iron** A deficiency reduces NK cell cytotoxicity, phagocytosis, and the bacterial killing capacity of cells called neutrophils.
- **Copper** A lack reduces the population of T cells and depresses the immune system.
- **Selenium** A deficiency decreases antibody production. Coupled with a shortage of vitamin E, it will also decrease the cytotoxic function of NK cells.
- **Pyridoxine** A lack of this B vitamin reduces antibody production and decreases the ability of lymphocytes to function.
- **Vitamin C** An antioxidant nutrient and antihistamine, vitamin C detoxifies histamine, which can depress the immune system.
- **Vitamin E** This antioxidant nutrient protects the lipid components of cells and is needed for selenium to function properly.

Learn the Benefits of Antioxidants and Phytochemicals

Protective elements such as antioxidant nutrients and phytochemicals are needed to enhance the immune system and protect the body from toxins and illness.

Antioxidant Nutrients: We have known for years that nutrients such as beta-carotene (a precursor to vitamin A), vitamins C and E, coenzyme Q$_{10}$, and selenium are free-radical scavengers. But scientists have recently discovered that many plant foods contain antioxidant properties in even higher concentrations. For example, powerful antioxidants such as the ellagic acid in raspberries, the proanthocyanidins in raisins, the glutathione in goat's and cow's milk, and the polyphenols in strawberries help to remove free radicals from the body.

Flavonoids: Flavonoids, like carotenoids, are a large family of pigments that turn food red, orange, and yellow. Those with antioxidant activity include rutin, quercetin, and the citrus flavones. Other pigments that neutralize free radicals are the proanthocyanidins, tannins, and anthocyanins—in other words, the pigments that impart red, blue, and purple color in foods. So as long as you eat a variety of colors, you can infuse your diet with an array of cancer-fighting nutrients!

Probiotics: We can protect the body from invaders that come in through the digestive tract by building microflora along the gut wall. Probiotics such as acidophilus and bifidophilus colonize in the digestive tract, forming a barrier that fends off toxins, bad bacteria, and fungus.

Black Tea: Black tea leaves offer antioxidant and immune-boosting potential. Regularly drinking black tea may lower your risk of ovarian cancer, according to a recent study reported in the *International Journal of Gynecological Cancer* (January 2007). In this study, black tea consumption was associated with a decline in ovarian cancer risk, and those consuming two or more cups daily experienced a 30 percent decline in risk.

Vitamin K Foods: Vitamin K may act as a toxin to cancer cells while not harming other cells. Add wheat bran flakes or cooked egg yolks to smoothies to introduce vitamin K.

Zinc Foods: Zinc is a mineral that is necessary for the production of white blood cells, which are the front line of defense against invaders such as viruses, bacteria, and yeasts. Zinc sources include almonds, peanuts, Brazil nuts, pecans, ginger root, pumpkin seeds, and wheat bran.

Vitamin B$_{12}$: Vitamin B$_{12}$ is involved in metabolism of protein fat and carbohydrates. It also aids in the formation of red blood cells, antibody production, and cell respiration and growth. Just 1 tablespoon per day of nutritional yeast supplies all of the B vitamins you need to improve your health and strengthen your natural defense systems.

Citrus Juice: Oranges contain phytochemicals in their skin that both protect against cells becoming cancerous and help fight existing cancers. The white part of the citrus peel contains bioflavanoids that inhibit procarcinogens such as those found in cigarette smoke and pesticides. Hesperetin, the most abundant bioflavonoid in orange juice, has been found to inhibit procarcinogens as well, significantly reducing the opportunity for them to be converted into carcinogens.

Strawberries: Strawberries are not only high in vitamin C and antioxidants but also contain the powerful cancer fighter ellagic acid.

Daily Cancer Fighter

This is a fresh twist on the classic V-8 drinks. The citrus brightens the flavor and the garlic gives it bite.

1 cup vegetable juice
2 garlic cloves, chopped
1 tablespoon flaxseed oil
1 teaspoon bran
1 tablespoon lemon juice
Freshly ground black pepper, to taste

Serves 1

Peppercorns are a rich source of potassium. Garlic is a natural antibiotic that helps stave off bacterial and viral infections, as it contains organosulfur compounds known to detoxify carcinogenic materials and block tumor growth. Lignin is a fiber found in the cell walls of plant foods such as wheat bran, flaxseeds, and some flax oils; lignin intake is associated with a lower incidence of cancer.

SERVING SIZE: 1 (278G)			
CALORIES: 190		**CALORIES FROM FAT: 120**	
	%DV*		%DV*
Total Fat 14g	22%	Sugars 10g	
Saturated Fat 1.5g	8%	Protein 2g	
Cholesterol 0mg	0%	Vitamin A	80%
Sodium 170mg	7%	Vitamin C	130%
Total Carbohydrate 15g	5%	Calcium	4%
Dietary Fiber 3g	12%	Iron	6%
*Percent Daily Values are based on a 2,000 calorie diet			

Banana Chocolate

Thick and creamy, this chocolate milkshake is powerful medicine.

1 cup milk
1 frozen peeled banana
1 tablespoon nutritional yeast
2 tablespoons unsweetened cocoa powder
Optional: 1 tablespoon sweetener

Serves 1

In addition to protein, dietary fiber, vitamins, and minerals, nutritional yeast contains functional and beneficial components such as beta-1,3 glucan, trehalose, mannan, and glutathione. Studies have show that these components have potential health benefits, such as improved immune response, reduction of cholesterol, and anti-cancer properties.

SERVING SIZE: 1 (375G)			
CALORIES: 290		**CALORIES FROM FAT: 80**	
	%DV*		%DV*
Total Fat 9g	14%	Sugars 25g	
Saturated Fat 4.5g	23%	Protein 13g	
Cholesterol 25mg	8%	Vitamin A	6%
Sodium 100mg	4%	Vitamin C	15%
Total Carbohydrate 51g	17%	Calcium	30%
Dietary Fiber 9g	37%	Iron	8%
*Percent Daily Values are based on a 2,000 calorie diet			

Cancer Killer

The rich apple flavor and light juice base of the Cancer Killer belies its tough, crime-fighting properties.

1 cup ice cubes
1 cup frozen apple juice concentrate
½ cup applesauce
1 teaspoon lecithin granules or liquid

Serves 2

Apples are an excellent source of quercetin, a commonly occurring flavanoid and powerful antioxidant that may be directly toxic to cancer cells. It also blocks the manufacture of the prostaglandin E2 series, which can depress the immune system. Additionally, the pectin found in apples has antimutagenic (anti-cancer) effects. These pectin polysaccharides interact directly with cells to protect them from mutagenic attack.

SERVING SIZE: ½ OF RECIPE (297G)			
CALORIES: 250		CALORIES FROM FAT: 10	
	%DV*		%DV*
Total Fat 1g	2%	Sugars 44g	
Saturated Fat 0g	0%	Protein 1g	
Cholesterol 0mg	0%	Vitamin A	0%
Sodium 50mg	2%	Vitamin C	6%
Total Carbohydrate 59g	20%	Calcium	4%
Dietary Fiber 1g	4%	Iron	8%
*Percent Daily Values are based on a 2,000 calorie diet			

Green Tea Garita

Cold and sweet like a margarita, but with all the potency of a Japanese ninja.

1 cup green tea
1 cup sparkling water
½ cup ice cubes
1 tablespoon xylitol

Serves 1

Aglycone, kaempferol, and myricetin are the flavonoids responsible for the potent cancer-fighting and antioxidant properties of Japanese green tea.

SERVING SIZE: 1 (592G)				
CALORIES: 0		**CALORIES FROM FAT: 0**		
	%DV*			%DV*
Total Fat 0g	0%	Sugars 0g		
Saturated Fat 0g	0%	Protein 0g		
Cholesterol 0mg	0%	Vitamin A		0%
Sodium 5mg	0%	Vitamin C		4%
Total Carbohydrate 0g	0%	Calcium		0%
Dietary Fiber 0g	0%	Iron		0%
*Percent Daily Values are based on a 2,000 calorie diet				

Immune Charger

This combination is very light and fresh, and surprisingly sweet, despite the carrots. It's a great way to get a daily influx of beta-carotene.

1 cup fresh carrot juice   ½ cup apple juice
1 garlic clove, sliced   1 teaspoon fresh lemon juice

Serves 1

Apples are a good source of the following: polyphenols, which are known for their antimicrobial action and infection-prevention abilities; glutathione, a potent antioxidant that helps prevent heart disease and cancer; and malic acid, a fruit acid that is a powerful binder of heavy metals such as cadmium and lead. Carrots are rich in the fat-soluble vitamins known as carotenoids that protect cells from environmental damage.

Clinical studies have found that ginger reduces the pain and swelling caused by osteoarthritis—that ginger relieved pain and/or swelling in 75 percent of arthritis patients.

SERVING SIZE: 1 (359G)			
CALORIES: 110		**CALORIES FROM FAT: 5**	
	%DV*		%DV*
Total Fat 0g	0%	Sugars 14g	
Saturated Fat 0g	0%	Protein 1g	
Cholesterol 0mg	0%	Vitamin A	100%
Sodium 120mg	5%	Vitamin C	25%
Total Carbohydrate 27g	9%	Calcium	6%
Dietary Fiber 0g	0%	Iron	2%
*Percent Daily Values are based on a 2,000 calorie diet			

Strawberries and Cream

This creamy strawberry shake is full of energy-supporting nutrients and protein. It can serve as a snack or meal replacement.

1 cup vanilla soymilk
½ cup plain yogurt
1 cup frozen strawberries

½ cup silken tofu
1 teaspoon vanilla extract

Serves 2

Strawberries are an excellent source of vitamin C, a known infection fighter. Yogurt has probiotics, which protect the gut from bacteria. And soy is an excellent protein source.

A powerful cancer-preventive agent in berries is ellagic acid, present in the tiny seeds of strawberries, raspberries, black raspberries, and blackberries. This compound has shown promising results in inhibiting tumor growth. Ellagic acid appears to act as an antioxidant, deactivating specific carcinogens and helping slow the reproduction of cancer cells.

SERVING SIZE: ½ OF RECIPE (312G)			
CALORIES: 180		**CALORIES FROM FAT: 30**	
	%DV*		%DV*
Total Fat 3.5g	5%	Sugars 16g	
Saturated Fat 0g	0%	Protein 12g	
Cholesterol 0mg	0%	Vitamin A	6%
Sodium 130mg	5%	Vitamin C	50%
Total Carbohydrate 25g	8%	Calcium	15%
Dietary Fiber 2g	8%	Iron	8%
*Percent Daily Values are based on a 2,000 calorie diet			

Banana Bran

This banana shake is velvety and sweet with just a hint of citrus.

1 cup yogurt
1 frozen peeled banana
2 tablespoons frozen orange juice concentrate
1 tablespoon flaxseed oil
1 tablespoon oat bran

Serves 1

Bran helps to remove waste or toxins from the body, which reduces stress on the immune system. Bananas are rich in vitamin B$_6$, which may help to prevent colorectal cancer in women, lower the risk of heart disease, and reduce the risk of breast cancer.

SERVING SIZE: 1 (394g)			
CALORIES: 300		**CALORIES FROM FAT: 5**	
	%DV*		%DV*
Total Fat 0.5g	1%	Sugars 45g	
Saturated Fat 0g	0%	Protein 17g	
Cholesterol 5mg	2%	Vitamin A	25%
Sodium 230mg	10%	Vitamin C	100%
Total Carbohydrate 61g	20%	Calcium	40%
Dietary Fiber 4g	16%	Iron	4%
*Percent Daily Values are based on a 2,000 calorie diet			

Kona Sunrise

This tropical shake is reminiscent of the exotic Hawaiian Islands.

1 cup organic soymilk
1 frozen peeled banana
½ cup mango nectar
½ cup fresh or canned pineapple
¼ cup toasted wheat germ

Serves 2

Copper is necessary for the proper functioning of the immune system, as it is part of superoxide dismutase, an enzyme necessary for protection from free radicals. Soybeans contain copper, and the wheat germ contains zinc, a mineral that needs to be a part of a copper-containing diet as the two minerals compete with each other.

SERVING SIZE: ½ OF RECIPE (305G)			
CALORIES: 230		**CALORIES FROM FAT: 35**	
	%DV*		%DV*
Total Fat 4g	6%	Sugars 25g	
Saturated Fat 0g	0%	Protein 10g	
Cholesterol 0mg	0%	Vitamin A	25%
Sodium 75mg	3%	Vitamin C	30%
Total Carbohydrate 42g	14%	Calcium	6%
Dietary Fiber 7g	28%	Iron	15%
*Percent Daily Values are based on a 2,000 calorie diet			

White Tea Icy

Try this if you are not a casual drinker of white tea and want to be turned on to something new and tasty.

1 cup white tea
½ cup ice cubes
1 tablespoon honey
Optional: 10 drops liquid folic acid

Serves 1

White tea leaves are grown in China and Japan and in the Darjeeling region of India. White tea has considerably less caffeine (15 mg per serving, compared to 40 mg for black tea and 20 mg for green), and many studies have found that white tea contains more immune-protecting antioxidants than green tea.

SERVING SIZE: 1 (376G)			
CALORIES: 70		**CALORIES FROM FAT: 0**	
	%DV*		%DV*
Total Fat 0g	0%	Sugars 16g	
Saturated Fat 0g	0%	Protein 0g	
Cholesterol 0mg	0%	Vitamin A	0%
Sodium 0mg	0%	Vitamin C	0%
Total Carbohydrate 17g	6%	Calcium	0%
Dietary Fiber 0g	0%	Iron	0%
*Percent Daily Values are based on a 2,000 calorie diet			

Katie's Feel Good Smoothie

A thick and hearty breakfast drink, this really will make you feel good for the rest of the day.

½ cup milk
½ cup orange juice
½ cup granola
½ cup yogurt
1 ripe bananas, peeled
Optional: ½ teaspoon vitamin C powder

Serves 2

When a vitamin C source is ingested along with whole grains such as those in granola, the phytic acid complex in the grain is broken down, freeing both the iron and the phytic acid. Phytic acid intake has been linked to a decreased cancer risk.

SERVING SIZE: ½ OF RECIPE (254G)			
CALORIES: 480		**CALORIES FROM FAT: 45**	
	%DV*		%DV*
Total Fat 5g	8%	Sugars 23g	
Saturated Fat 1g	5%	Protein 9g	
Cholesterol 10mg	3%	Vitamin A	10%
Sodium 90mg	4%	Vitamin C	60%
Total Carbohydrate 37g	12%	Calcium	20%
Dietary Fiber 3g	12%	Iron	4%
*Percent Daily Values are based on a 2,000 calorie diet			

Blueberry Baby

Frozen fruit gives this smoothie a delicious milkshake texture. This purple shake is infused with rich blueberry flavor.

1 cup frozen blueberries
1 cup apple juice
1 frozen peeled banana

Serves 1

The pigment that gives blueberries their rich blue color is among a group of powerful antioxidants called anthocyanins. Studies from Mount Sinai School of Medicine found that they contain cancer-protective ellagic acid and tannins that help prevent urinary tract infections, plus they may inhibit the growth of prostate, colon, and breast-cancer cells, as well as boost brain health and vision. Furthermore, the *Journal of the National Cancer Institute* found that increased intake of foods containing flavanoids, like those found in apples, have the potential to cut the risk of lung cancer in half.

SERVING SIZE: 1 (521G)			
CALORIES: 290		**CALORIES FROM FAT: 10**	
	%DV*		%DV*
Total Fat 1.5g	2%	Sugars 55g	
Saturated Fat 0g	0%	Protein 2g	
Cholesterol 0mg	0%	Vitamin A	2%
Sodium 0mg	0%	Vitamin C	30%
Total Carbohydrate 75g	25%	Calcium	2%
Dietary Fiber 7g	28%	Iron	6%
*Percent Daily Values are based on a 2,000 calorie diet			

Watermelon Lemonade

This light, refreshing melon slurpee has just a hint of lemon.

2 cups seedless watermelon pulp
1 cup sparkling water
1 cup ice cubes
1 teaspoon lemon juice

Serves 1

Watermelon is naturally rich in the cancer-fighting antioxidant lycopene, as well as vitamin C, carotenoids, and potassium.

SERVING SIZE: 1 (783G)			
CALORIES: 90		**CALORIES FROM FAT: 5**	
	%DV*		%DV*
Total Fat 0g	0%	Sugars 19g	
Saturated Fat 0g	0%	Protein 2g	
Cholesterol 0mg	0%	Vitamin A	35%
Sodium 15mg	1%	Vitamin C	45%
Total Carbohydrate 23g	8%	Calcium	6%
Dietary Fiber 1g	4%	Iron	4%
*Percent Daily Values are based on a 2,000 calorie diet			

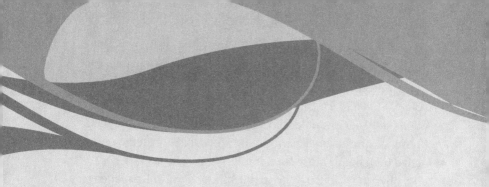

...Sleep Enhancers...

To this day, the processes behind sleep are still poorly understood by medical science. To the uninitiated, laying down and relaxing one's body might seem sufficient to allow a person to function the next day, even in the absence of true deep sleep. However, anyone who has suffered through sleep deprivation or insomnia knows how pervasively a lack of sleep affects his or her whole life. If the lack of rest itself were not sufficiently unpleasant, there is also the reduced ability to concentrate, the irritability, and a reduced immune response. There is also an unfortunate tendency for insomniacs to get trapped in drug dependency to meet their sleep needs. Luckily, there are some nutritional strategies that can help.

Strategies to Improve Sleep

Avoid Stimulants

One of the most important, and sometimes difficult, changes to enact is to reduce or remove all stimulants from the diet. Many insomniacs feel useless in the daytime without their coffee, tea, caffeine-rich sodas, or energy drinks. In mild episodes of sleep loss, avoiding caffeine after noon can help correct the problem.

But when sleep loss continues, a complete cessation of caffeine as well as other stimulants may be the only way to get back to normal sleep patterns. You will need to educate yourself on some of the less expected sources of stimulants and root those out as well. For example, chocolate has both caffeine and theobromine, and several pain medications have caffeine as an active ingredient. Most regular mild-stimulant users are actually physically addicted to them, and many will experience headaches and sometimes other symptoms on withdrawal. Be careful not to reintroduce caffeine in the guise of a headache medication.

Avoid Evening Supplements

Take supplements early in the day (before noon), as many, such as the B vitamins, may be stimulating at night.

Balance Your Hormones

Hormone cycles can affect sleeping patterns. Assist hormone balancing by avoiding endocrine disruptors such as plastics, perfumes, lawn chemicals, and harsh household-cleaning products. Use glass storage containers in the kitchen rather than plastic, natural oils rather than chemical perfumes, organic lawn-care methods and products, and natural household-cleaning products. Avoid hormones in the food supply, such as BGH in dairy products, by purchasing organic animal foods. Take probiotics, which help balance hormones as they metabolize nutrients such as the B vitamins, and make sure you're getting enough natural hormones from foods like licorice, soy, and flaxseeds, which contain phytoestrogens.

Increase Your Tryptophan

Tryptophan supports the production of serotonin, which enhances deep, restful sleep. Tryptophan also plays a significant role in the synthesis of the B vitamin niacin. Some foods that contain concentrated tryptophan are milk, cottage cheese, yogurt, seeds, nuts (especially cashews), mangoes, and papaya.

Increase Your Magnesium

The muscular and vascular relaxant magnesium is essential to proper sleep. Take it in supplement form or from foods such as nuts, seeds, and nut butters.

SLEEP-ENHANCING SMOOTHIE INGREDIENTS

- **Dairy** Foods that contain concentrated tryptophan, such as milk, cottage cheese, and yogurt, are delicious ingredients for sleep-inducing smoothies.
- **Fruits** Mangoes and papaya contain tryptophan.
- **Nuts** The tryptophan found in seeds and nuts, especially cashews, can be added to smoothies in the form of nut butters or ground nuts. Nuts and seeds are also good sources of magnesium and potassium, which remedy nighttime muscle cramps and twitching.
- **Tart cherries** Researchers at the University of Texas Health Science Center in San Antonio discovered that tart cherries contain significant quantities of melatonin. Melatonin is a hormone known for helping to regulate the body's internal clock and it appears to be key in regulating sleep cycles.

Sweet Dreams

This is a simple evening treat that's sweetly satisfying right before bed.

1 cup ice cubes
1 cup pitted tart cherries

Serves 1

Tart cherries contain significant amounts of melatonin—a hormone produced in the brain's pineal gland that has been credited with slowing the aging process, fighting insomnia, and warding off jet lag. It's also being studied as a potential treatment for cancer, depression, and other diseases and disorders.

SERVING SIZE: 1 (377G)			
CALORIES: 90		**CALORIES FROM FAT: 10**	
	%DV*		%DV*
Total Fat 1g	2%	Sugars 16g	
Saturated Fat 0g	0%	Protein 1g	
Cholesterol 0mg	0%	Vitamin A	0%
Sodium 10mg	0%	Vitamin C	8%
Total Carbohydrate 23g	8%	Calcium	2%
Dietary Fiber 3g	12%	Iron	0%
*Percent Daily Values are based on a 2,000 calorie diet			

Calming Cooler

This is an almond version of a Peanut Butter Cup shake (page 237). It represents a nice alternative for those with peanut allergies.

1 cup ice cubes
1 cup almond milk
2 tablespoons almond butter
½ teaspoon magnesium powder
¼ teaspoon vanilla extract

Serves 1

Magnesium is a universal relaxant. This mineral is responsible for relaxing muscles and blood vessels and provides a general feeling of well-being. Nuts such as almonds naturally contain magnesium.

SERVING SIZE: 1 (511G)			
CALORIES: 260		**CALORIES FROM FAT: 190**	
	%DV*		%DV*
Total Fat 21g	32%	Sugars 9g	
Saturated Fat 2g	10%	Protein 6g	
Cholesterol 0mg	0%	Vitamin A	10%
Sodium 300mg	13%	Vitamin C	0%
Total Carbohydrate 15g	5%	Calcium	30%
Dietary Fiber 2g	8%	Iron	8%
*Percent Daily Values are based on a 2,000 calorie diet			

Vanilla Malt

Malted shakes are nostalgic treats for many, reminiscent of the lazy summer days of childhood.

1 frozen peeled banana
1 cup milk
¼ cup nonfat dry milk powder
1 teaspoon vanilla extract
1 tablespoon malted milk powder

Serves 1

Milk and nonfat dry milk powder contain tryptophan, which is a precursor of serotonin and regarded as an effective sleep-inducing agent. Researchers at Boston State Hospital found that taking 1 gram of tryptophan can cut down the time it takes to fall asleep by ten to twenty minutes.

SERVING SIZE: 1 (404G)			
CALORIES: 410		**CALORIES FROM FAT: 90**	
	%DV*		%DV*
Total Fat 10g	15%	Sugars 45g	
Saturated Fat 6g	30%	Protein 18g	
Cholesterol 30mg	10%	Vitamin A	15%
Sodium 280mg	12%	Vitamin C	20%
Total Carbohydrate 63g	21%	Calcium	60%
Dietary Fiber 3g	12%	Iron	2%
*Percent Daily Values are based on a 2,000 calorie diet			

Vanilla Dream Shake

Dairy protein helps stabilize blood sugar for many hours, so let this dreamy vanilla shake set the stage for a restful night's sleep.

1 cup milk
½ cup plain yogurt
½ cup cottage cheese
1 frozen peeled banana
1 tablespoon flax meal (ground flaxseeds)
1 teaspoon vanilla extract

Serves 2

Yogurt and cottage cheese contain amino acids, which are the building blocks of protein. Amino acids are used by the body to produce neurotransmitters, such as the feel-good relaxers dopamine and serotonin.

SERVING SIZE: ½ OF RECIPE (301G)			
CALORIES: 230		**CALORIES FROM FAT: 60**	
	%DV*		%DV*
Total Fat 7g	11%	Sugars 19g	
Saturated Fat 4g	20%	Protein 16g	
Cholesterol 20mg	7%	Vitamin A	10%
Sodium 310mg	13%	Vitamin C	8%
Total Carbohydrate 28g	9%	Calcium	30%
Dietary Fiber 3g	12%	Iron	2%
*Percent Daily Values are based on a 2,000 calorie diet			

Creamy Cashew Clouds

This shake is light and fluffy like a cloud, and has an interesting, nutty flavor.

½ cup cashews, ground
1 cup milk
1 frozen peeled banana

Serves 2

Common antidepressant drugs work to increase the level of available serotonin in the brain. Naturally occurring tryptophan, however, can accomplish many of the same goals, as it is a key ingredient in the creation of serotonin. Unfortunately, the body can't make its own tryptophan, so we need to take it in through our diets. The magnesium in the nuts provides an additional relaxant, taking tension out of your muscles and preparing your body for rest.

SERVING SIZE: ½ OF RECIPE (215G)			
CALORIES: 320		**CALORIES FROM FAT: 180**	
	%DV*		%DV*
Total Fat 20g	31%	Sugars 14g	
Saturated Fat 5g	25%	Protein 10g	
Cholesterol 10mg	3%	Vitamin A	4%
Sodium 55mg	2%	Vitamin C	8%
Total Carbohydrate 30g	10%	Calcium	15%
Dietary Fiber 3g	12%	Iron	10%
*Percent Daily Values are based on a 2,000 calorie diet			

Tart Cherry Ginger

A sweet cherry flavor with a hint of spice makes this creamy shake a potent sleep-supporting dessert.

2 cups milk
1 teaspoon flaxseed oil
6 tablespoons protein powder
1½ tablespoons tart cherry juice concentrate
1 teaspoon ground ginger
2 cups frozen cherries

Serves 2

Cherries contain the potent antioxidant anthocyanins and have been shown to contain high levels of melatonin, the hormone said to induce sleep.

SERVING SIZE: ½ OF RECIPE (432G)			
CALORIES: 340		**CALORIES FROM FAT: 100**	
	%DV*		%DV*
Total Fat 12g	18%	Sugars 34g	
Saturated Fat 15g	25%	Protein 22g	
Cholesterol 45mg	15%	Vitamin A	30%
Sodium 150mg	6%	Vitamin C	4%
Total Carbohydrate 38g	13%	Calcium	40%
Dietary Fiber 3g	12%	Iron	98%
*Percent Daily Values are based on a 2,000 calorie diet			

Sweet Slumber

I use the Eden Organic Tart Cherry Juice Concentrate because it makes smoothies that are rich in flavor.

1 cup ice cubes
1 cup pitted tart cherries
2 tablespoons tart cherry concentrate
Optional: 1 teaspoon sweetener

Serves 2

Tart cherries contain significant amounts of melatonin, a hormone produced in the brain's pineal gland that is said to induce sleep.

SERVING SIZE: ½ OF RECIPE (209G)				
CALORIES: 90		**CALORIES FROM FAT: 5**		
	%DV*			%DV*
Total Fat 0.5g	1%	Sugars 19g		
Saturated Fat 0g	0%	Protein 1g		
Cholesterol 0mg	0%	Vitamin A		0%
Sodium 30mg	1%	Vitamin C		4%
Total Carbohydrate 23g	8%	Calcium		2%
Dietary Fiber 2g	8%	Iron		2%
*Percent Daily Values are based on a 2,000 calorie diet				

Banana Nutmeg Smoothie

Nutmeg and vanilla are comfort flavors for many people. Just smelling these warm spices is enough to trigger the neuro-transmitters that support relaxation.

1 cup milk
½ cup cottage cheese
1 frozen peeled banana
2 tablespoons peanut butter
¼ teaspoon grated nutmeg
¼ teaspoon vanilla extract

Serves 2

Milk, cottage cheese, and nuts support the production of melatonin, the sleep-inducing hormone. Nuts also contain magnesium, a universal muscle relaxant.

SERVING SIZE: ½ OF RECIPE (255G)			
CALORIES: 270		**CALORIES FROM FAT: 130**	
	%DV*		%DV*
Total Fat 15g	23%	Sugars 16g	
Saturated Fat 5g	25%	Protein 15g	
Cholesterol 20mg	7%	Vitamin A	6%
Sodium 330mg	14%	Vitamin C	8%
Total Carbohydrate 25g	8%	Calcium	20%
Dietary Fiber 3g	12%	Iron	2%
*Percent Daily Values are based on a 2,000 calorie diet			

Dreamer's Delight

The herbal base in Dreamer's Delight is sweet enough as is, so it is perfect for those who are trying to avoid sugar or cut back on calories. Bengal Spice is a Celestial Seasonings tea blend with lots of cinnamon, chicory, carob, and vanilla.

1 cup steeped Bengal Spice tea
½ cup ice cubes
¼ cup milk
Optional: 1 tablespoon honey

Serves 1

Raw, unpasteurized honey has not been heat-treated and is believed to contain natural antibacterial agents. Milk contains tryptophan and melatonin.

SERVING SIZE: 1 (416G)			
CALORIES: 35		**CALORIES FROM FAT: 20**	
	%DV*		%DV*
Total Fat 2g	3%	Sugars 3g	
Saturated Fat 1g	5%	Protein 2g	
Cholesterol 5mg	2%	Vitamin A	2%
Sodium 30mg	1%	Vitamin C	0%
Total Carbohydrate 3g	1%	Calcium	8%
Dietary Fiber 0g	0%	Iron	0%
*Percent Daily Values are based on a 2,000 calorie diet			

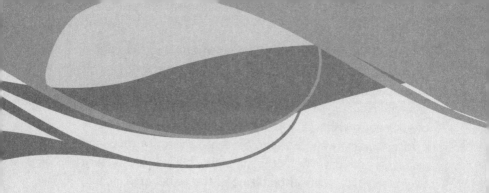

...Stress and Blood Pressure Reducers...

High blood pressure is a major risk factor in heart disease, which is the leading cause of death in the United States. Those with hypertension, even without other symptoms, have a higher risk of developing heart disease or stroke. The door to both stress and high blood pressure is thrown wide open when certain nutrient deficiencies are present.

We should all take measures to prevent high blood pressure because it is so frightfully common and frequently remains undiagnosed. It causes no pain and gives us no warning as it quietly damages blood vessels, which increases the risk for stroke, kidney disease, and congestive heart failure. Diet can be a powerful remedy to high blood pressure, and thanks to the vast amount of research at our fingertips we have discovered several natural functional foods that can help prevent and reverse this disorder. Increasing the fruits and vegetables in our diets while reducing animal products, for example, can drastically lessen your vulnerability to a stroke or heart attack, as many studies have found that vegetarians have lower blood pressure than nonvegetarians.

The Nutrition Committee of the American Heart Association estimates that by lowering diastolic blood pressure by just 2 millimeters, the risk of stroke is lowered by as much as 15 percent and heart disease risk by 6 percent. Losing just 10 percent of your body weight, if you are overweight, also lowers blood pressure dramatically. So aim for eight servings of fruits and vegetables per day. Five is the minimum, but if you can reach twelve servings, you will be taking in the actual amount that most of the studies recommend. A serving is about ½ cup.

Fruits and vegetables are rich in potassium, which also helps lower blood pressure. Most Americans lack this important mineral. A recent study found that only 10 percent of men and 1 percent of women get the recommended 4.7 grams a day. Fruits and vegetables are also rich in fiber, vitamins, minerals, and phytochemicals that help to stabilize blood pressure. In two major diet trials, increased intake of fruits and vegetables resulted in substantial drops in blood pressure. In fact, diet is so effective in controlling blood pressure that even those who are currently taking medication are often able to reduce or eliminate their regimen once they've made basic dietary changes.

Likewise, too much cholesterol reduces the flexibility of the blood vessels over time owing to the formation of plaque (arteriosclerosis), which can also contribute to high blood pressure. Laboratory tests suggest that some berries may reduce the buildup of LDL (low-density lipoprotein) cholesterol, a contributor to heart disease, stroke, and atherosclerosis. Raspberries were tested as having the second highest LDL inhibitory effect. Interestingly, the anthocyanin content (believed to be a protective antioxidant) of raspberries *increases* in storage, thus increasing their antioxidant value over time.

Key Smoothie Ingredients

Omega-3 Fatty Acids

Alpha-linolenic acid promotes vascular health. Add ground flaxseed or flaxseed oil, pumpkin seeds, and walnuts to your smoothies to infuse them with these rich fats, which are necessary for healthy brain and circulatory activity.

Electrolyte Supplements

The electrolyte minerals potassium, magnesium, sodium, calcium, and chloride are needed to conduct electricity through our bodies. These minerals help move the electrical current through our hearts to help them beat in rhythm. Fruits and vegetables contain these minerals in varying degrees. Liquid or powdered electrolyte products are also widely available and blend well into smoothies.

Soluble and Insoluble Fiber

Soluble and insoluble fiber removes toxic waste and cholesterol from the body. Toxins deplete nutrients, so it is important to keep toxin loads low. Soluble-fiber food sources include pectin from apples and pears, rice bran, and citrus fruits. Insoluble-fiber sources include fruit, wheat bran, rolled oats, and ground flaxseed.

Magnesium

Magnesium helps to lower and control blood pressure by relaxing blood vessels and allowing the blood to move more easily throughout the body. Some good magnesium food sources are avocados, dark chocolate, pumpkin seeds, sunflower seeds, Brazil nuts, and almonds.

Calcium

This mineral stimulates muscles and contracts blood vessels. Calcium deficiency can cause nerve sensitivity, muscle twitching, irritability, and insomnia. Make sure to eat enough milk, yogurt, and cheese to keep your calcium blood levels at an appropriate level.

Vitamin C

Vitamin C is a water-soluble vitamin that helps to relax the blood vessels by making them more flexible. Food sources include tangerines, oranges, kiwi, and strawberries.

Potassium

Studies have shown that participants receiving potassium supplements often experience a significant reduction in blood pressure. Food sources are raisins, bananas, pomegranates, and avocados.

Wheat Germ

Wheat germ is wildly beneficial for its excess store of vitamin E and Coenzyme Q_{10} (CoQ10). Recent studies have shown that the antioxidant properties of Coenzyme Q_{10} benefit the body, the brain, and the heart muscle, and supplemental C0Q10 is now being used to protect the brain from neurodegenerative disease like Parkinson's and from the damaging side effects of a transient ischemic attack (stroke).

Red Grapefruit

Red grapefruit's antioxidants decrease total cholesterol and low-density lipoprotein (LDL) cholesterol, as well as unhealthy, artery-clogging triglycerides. The natural chemicals that occur in grapefruit are known to interact with certain medications—sometimes adversely—so people on prescription medication should take caution and consult with their doctor or pharmacist before consuming grapefruit products.

Cocoa

Flavanols present in certain cocoas have sufficient activity on vascular nitric oxide to influence blood pressure control.

Phytochemicals

Resveratrol: The phytochemical resveratrol, which is found in grapes, acts as a blood thinner and relaxes blood vessels.

Berries: Blackberries, blueberries, raspberries, cherries, and cranberries are excellent sources of antioxidants and anti-inflammatory phytochemicals, including polyphenols and anthocyanins. These help lower blood pressure as well as cholesterol.

Polyphenols: Polyphenols, which are found in red wines, green tea, apples, berries, pomegranates, and dark chocolate, have potent antioxidant properties and a host of documented benefits against cancer, heart disease, vision disorders, allergies, viral infections, and more.

Watermelon Pomegranate

This juicy icy is sweet, but the tart pomagranate gives it a little kick, as well as upping the health factor by several notches.

1 cup ice cubes
1 cup seedless
    watermelon

1 cup sparkling water
¼ cup pomegranate juice
1 teaspoon electrolyte powder

Serves 2

Pomegranates are a rich source of antioxidants. The Preventive Medicine Research Institute issued a report regarding the cardiovascular benefits of pomegranate. According to them, the juice contains antioxidants such as soluble polyphenols, tannins, and anthocyanins that protect the heart from atherosclerosis. The researchers concluded that daily consumption of pomegranate juice may actually improve stress-induced heart disease. The watermelon in this recipe provides heart-healthy carotenoids and the electrolyte powder contains the minerals necessary for electrical regulation of the heartbeat.

SERVING SIZE: ½ OF RECIPE (346G)			
CALORIES: 40		**CALORIES FROM FAT: 0**	
	%DV*		%DV*
Total Fat 0g	0%	Sugars 9g	
Saturated Fat 0g	0%	Protein 1g	
Cholesterol 0mg	0%	Vitamin A	8%
Sodium 10mg	0%	Vitamin C	10%
Total Carbohydrate 10g	3%	Calcium	8%
Dietary Fiber 0g	0%	Iron	2%
*Percent Daily Values are based on a 2,000 calorie diet			

Vaso Perfection

This creamy, dreamy combination of nuts and vanilla is so delicious you'll begin to relax on the first sip. The nutrients for stress and blood pressure are pretty powerful, too!

1 frozen peeled banana
1 cup ice cubes
1 cup milk
½ cup yogurt
2 tablespoons almond butter
1 teaspoon vanilla extract
1 teaspoon wheat germ
1 teaspoon flaxseed oil

Serves 2

The banana provides potassium, the nuts magnesium, the milk calcium, and the flax oil EFAs. The yogurt contains probiotics, which support digestion and protect against bacteria, viruses, and fungal infections. New research shows that probiotics may relieve intestinal disorders triggered by stress.

SERVING SIZE: ½ OF RECIPE (378G)			
CALORIES: 290		**CALORIES FROM FAT: 140**	
	%DV*		%DV*
Total Fat 16g	25%	Sugars 18g	
Saturated Fat 3.5g	18%	Protein 11g	
Cholesterol 15mg	5%	Vitamin A	8%
Sodium 180mg	8%	Vitamin C	8%
Total Carbohydrate 28g	9%	Calcium	30%
Dietary Fiber 2g	8%	Iron	4%
*Percent Daily Values are based on a 2,000 calorie diet			

Cherries and Cream

Creamy and rich in cherry flavor, this milky concoction will leave you blissful.

1 cup milk
1 cup frozen pitted cherries
¼ cup cottage cheese
Optional: 1 tablespoon flaxseed

Serves 2

Cherries are rich in the polyphenols and anthocyanins that help lower blood pressure, as well as cholesterol, when eaten regularly.

SERVING SIZE: ½ OF RECIPE (228G)			
CALORIES: 130		**CALORIES FROM FAT: 50**	
	%DV*		%DV*
Total Fat 5g	8%	Sugars 14g	
Saturated Fat 3g	15%	Protein 8g	
Cholesterol 15mg	5%	Vitamin A	15%
Sodium 150mg	6%	Vitamin C	2%
Total Carbohydrate 15g	5%	Calcium	15%
Dietary Fiber 1g	4%	Iron	2%
*Percent Daily Values are based on a 2,000 calorie diet			

Purple Power

Use frozen Concord grape juice concentrate and water for a thicker version of this smoothie. The punchy flavor of grapes is always fresh and invigorating.

2 cups ice cubes
1 cup sparkling water
¼ cup frozen purple grape juice concentrate

Serves 2

The phytochemical resveratrol is found in grapes and acts as a blood thinner and blood-vessel relaxant.

SERVING SIZE: ½ OF RECIPE (391G)			
CALORIES: 60		**CALORIES FROM FAT: 0**	
	%DV*		%DV*
Total Fat 0g	0%	Sugars 16g	
Saturated Fat 0g	0%	Protein 0g	
Cholesterol 0mg	0%	Vitamin A	0%
Sodium 15mg	1%	Vitamin C	50%
Total Carbohydrate 16g	5%	Calcium	2%
Dietary Fiber 0g	0%	Iron	0%
*Percent Daily Values are based on a 2,000 calorie diet			

Cherry Icy

Use your favorite dark berries in this recipe, as they are all delicious.

1 cup ice cubes
1 cup sparkling water
2 cups frozen pitted dark cherries
1 teaspoon sweetener
1 tablespoon cherry juice concentrate

Serves 2

The Harvard Medical School, Georgetown Medical Center, and the University of California at Davis are in agreement: anthocyanin-rich berries have potent cardiovascular protective effects. These include cherries, wild blueberries, strawberries, wild bilberries, cranberries, elderberries, and raspberries.

SERVING SIZE: ½ OF RECIPE (405G)			
CALORIES: 110		**CALORIES FROM FAT: 5**	
	%DV*		%DV*
Total Fat 0.5g	1%	Sugars 22g	
Saturated Fat 0g	0%	Protein 2g	
Cholesterol 0mg	0%	Vitamin A	25%
Sodium 20mg	1%	Vitamin C	4%
Total Carbohydrate 26g	9%	Calcium	4%
Dietary Fiber 3g	12%	Iron	6%
*Percent Daily Values are based on a 2,000 calorie diet			

Creamy Peach Smoothie

Peach nectar has a much richer flavor than peach juice and even many fresh peaches.

1 frozen peeled banana
½ cup milk
½ cup peach nectar
½ cup yogurt
1 teaspoon nutritional yeast

Serves 2

Nutritional yeast contains B vitamins. Daily intake of the vitamins B_6, B_{12}, and folic acid help to keep homocysteine levels down. Many studies indicate that high levels of homocysteine contribute to cardiovascular disease.

SERVING SIZE: ½ OF RECIPE (239G)			
CALORIES: 160		**CALORIES FROM FAT: 20**	
	%DV*		%DV*
Total Fat 2g	3%	Sugars 23g	
Saturated Fat 1g	5%	Protein 7g	
Cholesterol 10mg	3%	Vitamin A	10%
Sodium 85mg	4%	Vitamin C	15%
Total Carbohydrate 30g	10%	Calcium	20%
Dietary Fiber 2g	8%	Iron	2%
*Percent Daily Values are based on a 2,000 calorie diet			

Almond Elixir

Almonds have a lighter flavor than peanuts and are delicious in smoothies.

1 cup ice cubes
½ cup almond milk
1 tablespoon almond butter
1 teaspoon flaxseed oil

Serves 1

According to researchers at the University of Toronto, just one handful of almonds a day reduces LDL (bad cholesterol) by nearly 5 percent, and two handfuls cut LDL by 10 percent. Essential fatty acids found in flaxseed oil, such as GLA, also help reduce the unhealthy LDL and raise the beneficial HDL levels.

SERVING SIZE: 1 (378G)			
CALORIES: 170		**CALORIES FROM FAT: 140**	
	%DV*		%DV*
Total Fat 15g	23%	Sugars 4g	
Saturated Fat 1.5g	8%	Protein 3g	
Cholesterol 0mg	0%	Vitamin A	6%
Sodium 160mg	7%	Vitamin C	0%
Total Carbohydrate 7g	2%	Calcium	15%
Dietary Fiber 1g	4%	Iron	4%
*Percent Daily Values are based on a 2,000 calorie diet			

Blueberry Whip

This light and frothy whip is the perfect base for supplements such as probiotics, protein powder, flaxseed oil, and liquid calcium.

1 cup blueberry juice
1 cup fresh blueberries
½ cup ice cubes
½ cup milk

Serves 1

Blueberries and blueberry juice contain powerful cardio-vascular-protecting antioxidants and phytochemicals such as anthocyanins, ellagic acid, catechins, and resveratrol.

SERVING SIZE: 1 (641G)			
CALORIES: 300		**CALORIES FROM FAT: 40**	
	%DV*		%DV*
Total Fat 4.5g	7%	Sugars 44g	
Saturated Fat 2g	8%	Protein 6g	
Cholesterol 10mg	3%	Vitamin A	4%
Sodium 75mg	3%	Vitamin C	25%
Total Carbohydrate 48g	16%	Calcium	20%
Dietary Fiber 4g	16%	Iron	8%
*Percent Daily Values are based on a 2,000 calorie diet			

Lemon Drop

This sweet, citrus cocktail shimmers with bright flavor.

2 cups sparkling water
½ cup seedless grapes
2 tablespoons orange juice concentrate
1 tablespoon lemon juice
1 teaspoon electrolyte powder
1 teaspoon honey

Serves 1

Electrolyte minerals are essential to carry electrical currents through the body. When we are low in these minerals—calcium, magnesium, potassium, and sodium—we can become fatigued, have an irregular heartbeat, feel depressed, or experience muscle weakness. Replacing these minerals instantly corrects the problem, giving us more energy.

SERVING SIZE: 1 (611G)			
CALORIES: 140		**CALORIES FROM FAT: 0**	
	%DV*		%DV*
Total Fat 0g	0%	Sugars 31g	
Saturated Fat 0g	0%	Protein 1g	
Cholesterol 0mg	0%	Vitamin A	4%
Sodium 10mg	0%	Vitamin C	110%
Total Carbohydrate 35g	12%	Calcium	8%
Dietary Fiber 1g	4%	Iron	2%
*Percent Daily Values are based on a 2,000 calorie diet			

Peanut Butter Dream

Creamy and decadent, this thick treat is rich in cocoa and peanut butter flavor.

1 cup ice cubes
½ cup milk
½ cup cottage cheese
¼ cup peanut butter
2 tablespoons unsweetened cocoa powder
1 tablespoon wheat germ

Serves 2

Here, wheat germ offers CoQ10 while the cottage cheese provides concentrated protein, and the peanuts EFAs. Epichatechin is a flavanol found in cocoa and is associated with healthy circulation and cardiovascular function.

SERVING SIZE: ½ OF RECIPE (277G)			
CALORIES: 300		**CALORIES FROM FAT: 190**	
	%DV*		%DV*
Total Fat 21g	32%	Sugars 8g	
Saturated Fat 5g	25%	Protein 18g	
Cholesterol 15mg	5%	Vitamin A	4%
Sodium 390mg	16%	Vitamin C	0%
Total Carbohydrate 16g	5%	Calcium	15%
Dietary Fiber 4g	16%	Iron	6%
*Percent Daily Values are based on a 2,000 calorie diet			

Tart Cherry Tropical Cooler

This sorbet is a sweet mix of fresh tropical flavors with a tart cherry finish.

2 cups milk
2 cups mixed tropical fruit (melon, pineapple, strawberry, mango)
1 teaspoon flaxseed oil
6 tablespoons protein powder
1½ tablespoons tart cherry juice concentrate

Serves 2

Tart cherries contain natural anti-inflammatory compounds, called anthocyanins. Research at Michigan State University indicates that these compounds protect artery walls from plaque buildup and heart disease.

SERVING SIZE: ½ OF RECIPE (503G)			
CALORIES: 340		**CALORIES FROM FAT: 100**	
	%DV*		%DV*
Total Fat 12g	18%	Sugars 31g	
Saturated Fat 5g	25%	Protein 22g	
Cholesterol 45mg	15%	Vitamin A	6%
Sodium 150mg	6%	Vitamin C	220%
Total Carbohydrate 38g	13%	Calcium	45%
Dietary Fiber 5g	20%	Iron	8%
*Percent Daily Values are based on a 2,000 calorie diet			

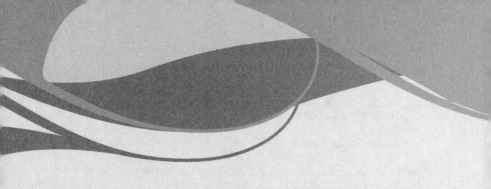

...Blood Sugar Stabilizers...

Blood sugar is the fuel that feeds our brains and muscles. When the sugar level in our bloodstream drops dramatically, it creates a state of low blood sugar. Those who have experienced this imbalance know how awful it feels. Some people experience panic, feel sweaty and shaky, and are weak and a little light-headed or confused. Low blood sugar is also known as *hypoglycemia* and is generally caused by too little food and is triggered by exercise or stimulants such as coffee.

Diabetes, on the other hand, is a condition in which either the body does not produce enough insulin or the cells of the body become resistant to insulin. When the pancreas slows down insulin production, there is not enough insulin to grab up the sugar in the bloodstream and carry it into the cells. This results in high blood sugar or *hyperglycemia*. When this happens over a period of time or the bloodstream sugar level spikes dramatically, your doctor may recommend that you take additional insulin. The dietary goal here is to match the amount of insulin in your body with the calories you have ingested, specifically carbohydrates. This serves to stabilize blood sugar levels. However, it is also possible to help stabilize your blood sugar levels through diet.

Strategies for Stabilizing Blood Sugar

Reduce Sugar Intake

Eating too much sugar causes a spike of sugar in the blood-stream, which triggers the pancreas to react by pumping out high levels of insulin. For a diabetic whose body cannot make insulin, this crisis can be averted by taking a prescribed insulin shot. However, for the rest of us, the pancreas often overre-sponds and drops blood sugar lower than normal, resulting in the low blood sugar that leaves a person weak and listless. The roller-coaster continues from there.

Therefore, one of the main dietary approaches for blood sugar control is simply to reduce the amount of sugar you eat, especially simple sugars such as cane sugar, honey, maple syrup, corn syrup, and beet sugars. Minimizing consumption of refined carbohydrates, which are chains of sugars, can also improve the situation; these break down quickly in the diges-tive tract, loading the system with sugar. Although noncaloric synthetic sweeteners may at first glance seem like good options, chemically produced sweeteners such as aspartame (NutraSweet), saccharin, acesulfame K (SweetOne or Sunette), and sucralose (Splenda) have all been linked to serious condi-tions such as bladder cancer, neurological problems, and arthritis.

Choose sweeteners that are natural, but low in calories, such as the sugar-alcohol xylitol or herbal sweeteners such as stevia and chicory, or Low Han Fruit.

Increase Protein Intake

Increase protein in the diet, preferably from both animal and plant sources. How much protein do we need? The recom-mended intake of protein is generally 15 to 25 percent of your total caloric intake. Age, gender, and body weight determine an individual's caloric needs, and protein needs are calculated as a percentage of total calories consumed each day. Below is a chart that lists protein needs based on caloric intake.

PROTEIN NEEDS BASED ON DAILY CALORIC INTAKE	
1,200 calories/day	45–75 grams protein
1,500 calories/day	56–93 grams protein
2,000 calories/day	75–125 grams protein
2,500 calories/day	93–156 grams protein
3,000 calories/day	112–187 grams protein

In general, your body needs only .36 grams of protein per pound of body weight (although infants, children, athletes, and pregnant and nursing women may require more). To calculate the exact amount of protein you need, multiply your ideal weight by .36. This will give you your optimum daily protein requirement in grams.

Animal Sources of Protein: Protein from animals that work well as smoothie ingredients are milk, cottage cheese, nonfat dry milk powder, whey-based protein powders, and yogurt.

Plant Sources of Protein: Protein from plant sources is a healthy choice because it does not contain cholesterol and does contain fiber, which animal foods do not. Many plant-based protein foods, such as nuts, seeds, nut butters, and avocados, also contain essential fatty acids. Soy products such as tofu, soy yogurt, and soymilk are also excellent smoothie additions.

Increase Fiber

Fiber is found in plant foods such as vegetables, fruits, grains, and legumes. Legumes are beans, peas, and lentils that contain soluble and insoluble fiber. Vegetables, grains, and legumes all have low sugar content. Oats and barley offer a type of fiber called beta-glucans, and legumes contain a type of fiber called arabinose. When fruit is eaten whole rather than processed, it is rich in soluble fiber such as pectin, which slows the release of the fruit sugar into the system, thus reducing its glycemic load.

Increase Water

One of the key aspects of blood sugar control is to stay well hydrated, which keeps the blood, including sugar, diluted and moving through the body.

Sparkling Water: Mineral waters such as San Pellegrino, Perrier, and San Faustino are free of sugar and add a little bubble to smoothies. If you have a hard time drinking enough water each day, consider adding more water or ice to your smoothies.

Ice: Use filtered water for making ice so your ice cubes won't taste like chlorine or chloramine, which are found in most tap water.

Eat Breakfast

Give your body fuel the first thing in the morning. For those taking insulin, drinking the same morning smoothie each day will make it easier to control your blood sugar. Just be sure that your smoothie has roughly the same number of calories as the breakfast you are replacing. Add ingredients such as dried fruit, frozen berries, or almond butter to increase the calories, if needed.

Smoothie Ingredients for Stabilizing Blood Sugar

Nuts and Seeds

Chromium is a trace mineral that our bodies use to assist in the transportation of sugar from the blood to the cells. When we are deficient in this nutrient, sugar builds up in the blood, causing high blood sugar levels yet leaving our cells starved. When this happens, our brains signal us to eat sugar. These sugar cravings are a warning sign that there may be a chromium deficiency. To avoid chromium deficiency, increase chromium-containing foods such as nuts, seeds, and nut butter.

Dark Berries

Dark berries such as blackberries, cherries, blueberries, raspberries, and strawberries are low on the glycemic index and are great choices for smoothies to help control blood sugar.

Oats and Oat Bran

These are good sources of beta-glucan, a soluble fiber that can help keep your glucose levels in normal range by decreasing how quickly food leaves the stomach.

Magnesium

Those with diabetes and hypoglycemia often test low for the mineral magnesium. Signs of deficiency include jumpiness, foot tapping or other nervous habits, muscle tension, high blood pressure, and constipation. Food sources include nuts, seeds, nut butters, and cocoa.

Banana Oat Smoothie

My dad, Tony, makes his morning smoothie with a cereal grain such as rolled oats or a lightly sweetened granola to add fiber. The texture is surprisingly delightful!

1 cup milk
¼ cup oatmeal or granola
1 banana, peeled
2 tablespoons chopped nuts
1 teaspoon flaxseed oil

Serves 2

Fiber slows down the absorption of carbohydrates, thus regulating blood sugar levels. Specific components of fiber, such as beta-glucans found in oats and barley, are especially helpful for blood sugar regulation for those with hypoglycemia or diabetes.

SERVING SIZE: ½ OF RECIPE (197G)			
CALORIES: 220		**CALORIES FROM FAT: 100**	
	%DV*		%DV*
Total Fat 11g	17%	Sugars 15g	
Saturated Fat 3g	15%	Protein 7g	
Cholesterol 10mg	3%	Vitamin A	4%
Sodium 55mg	2%	Vitamin C	8%
Total Carbohydrate 25g	8%	Calcium	15%
Dietary Fiber 3g	12%	Iron	4%
*Percent Daily Values are based on a 2,000 calorie diet			

Chocolate Macadanilla

Macadamia nuts and vanilla seem to have been made for each other. Use unsweetened dark cocoa for the greatest health benefits, and sweeten to taste with a low-calorie but natural sweetener such as xylitol, stevia, or Just Like Sugar.

1 cup milk
3 tablespoons unsweetened cocoa powder
2 tablespoons macadamia nut butter
2 teaspoons protein powder
1 teaspoon xylitol
1 tablespoon minced vanilla bean or 1 teaspoon extract

Serves 2

Cocoa is rich in antioxidant flavonoids called flavonols, which include procyanidins, epicatechins, and catechins. Studies have shown that people with high blood levels of flavonoids have lower risk of developing type 2 diabetes.

SERVING SIZE: ½ OF RECIPE (149G)			
CALORIES: 220		**CALORIES FROM FAT: 150**	
	%DV*		%DV*
Total Fat 17g	26%	Sugars 6g	
Saturated Fat 4.5g	23%	Protein 8g	
Cholesterol 15mg	5%	Vitamin A	2%
Sodium 50mg	2%	Vitamin C	0%
Total Carbohydrate 13g	4%	Calcium	15%
Dietary Fiber 3g	12%	Iron	4%
*Percent Daily Values are based on a 2,000 calorie diet			

akfast Shake

Cinnamon gives this smoothie a spicy personality. Blend the yogurt and the granola first. Then add the banana, milk, and cinnamon.

½ cup yogurt
½ cup granola
1 frozen peeled banana
½ cup milk
1 teaspoon ground cinnamon

Serves 2

Cinnamon helps prevent heart disease and type 2 diabetes. Owing to its antioxidant properties, cinnamon also helps people use the hormone insulin in their bodies more efficiently.

SERVING SIZE: ½ OF RECIPE (193G)			
CALORIES: 200		**CALORIES FROM FAT: 40**	
	%DV*		%DV*
Total Fat 4.5g	7%	Sugars 17g	
Saturated Fat 1g	5%	Protein 8g	
Cholesterol 10mg	3%	Vitamin A	8%
Sodium 90mg	4%	Vitamin C	10%
Total Carbohydrate 32g	11%	Calcium	20%
Dietary Fiber 4g	16%	Iron	6%
*Percent Daily Values are based on a 2,000 calorie diet			

Açaí Icy

A juicy slurpee infused with color and even richer in flavor.

1 cup ice cubes
½ cup blueberries
½ cup açaí juice
½ cup apple juice

Serves 2

The juices in this icy are all rich in antioxidants that support proper liver function, which is necessary for blood sugar control.

SERVING SIZE: ½ OF RECIPE (281G)			
CALORIES: 80		**CALORIES FROM FAT: 0**	
	%DV*		%DV*
Total Fat 0g	0%	Sugars 16g	
Saturated Fat 0g	0%	Protein 1g	
Cholesterol 0mg	0%	Vitamin A	0%
Sodium 15mg	1%	Vitamin C	8%
Total Carbohydrate 21g	7%	Calcium	2%
Dietary Fiber 1g	4%	Iron	2%
*Percent Daily Values are based on a 2,000 calorie diet			

Blackberry Cream

The next time you have blackberries, imagine how perfect they'd be in a thick, creamy smoothie. Then go make one! This delicious shake is rich in flavor with just a hint of citrus.

½ cup milk
¼ cup blackberries
1 frozen peeled banana
2 teaspoons lemon juice
2 tablespoons cottage cheese or yogurt

Serves 1

Cottage cheese is loaded with protein (3.5 g per tablespoon) and blends so well you'll think you're drinking cream. Protein often satisfies the body's energy needs better than sugar and will take you off the cravings roller-coaster.

SERVING SIZE: 1 (316G)			
CALORIES: 230		**CALORIES FROM FAT: 50**	
	%DV*		%DV*
Total Fat 6g	9%	Sugars 25g	
Saturated Fat 3g	15%	Protein 9g	
Cholesterol 15mg	5%	Vitamin A	6%
Sodium 150mg	6%	Vitamin C	25%
Total Carbohydrate 40g	13%	Calcium	20%
Dietary Fiber 5g	20%	Iron	4%
*Percent Daily Values are based on a 2,000 calorie diet			

Cherrilicious

This is a light whip that's not too sweet, but fairly filling and pleasantly textured.

1 cup milk
1 cup frozen pitted cherries
½ cup vanilla yogurt

Serves 2

Michigan State University researchers recently isolated several anthocyanins from cornelian cherries, testing them on insulin-producing pancreatic cells taken from rodents. The cells significantly increased their insulin production when exposed to the anthocyanins.

SERVING SIZE: ½ OF RECIPE (256G)			
CALORIES: 140		**CALORIES FROM FAT: 45**	
	%DV*		%DV*
Total Fat 5g	8%	Sugars 16g	
Saturated Fat 3g	15%	Protein 7g	
Cholesterol 15mg	5%	Vitamin A	20%
Sodium 90mg	4%	Vitamin C	4%
Total Carbohydrate 18g	6%	Calcium	25%
Dietary Fiber 1g	4%	Iron	2%
*Percent Daily Values are based on a 2,000 calorie diet			

Blueberry Citrus Blast

Lime juice brightens the flavor of berry drinks!

1 cup ice cubes
1 cup milk
1 cup frozen blueberries
2 tablespoons nonfat dry milk
2 teaspoons lime juice
1 tablespoon nutritional yeast
Optional: 1 teaspoon xylitol

Serves 2

Nutritional yeast is not only an excellent source of B vitamins but also of chromium. Chromium is a trace mineral that works to stabilize glucose levels in the blood by helping glucose get into cells, where it can be used as fuel and brain food.

SERVING SIZE: ½ OF RECIPE (329G)			
CALORIES: 130		**CALORIES FROM FAT: 40**	
	%DV*		%DV*
Total Fat 4.5g	7%	Sugars 14g	
Saturated Fat 2.5g	13%	Protein 7g	
Cholesterol 15mg	5%	Vitamin A	6%
Sodium 80mg	3%	Vitamin C	6%
Total Carbohydrate 18g	6%	Calcium	20%
Dietary Fiber 2g	8%	Iron	2%
*Percent Daily Values are based on a 2,000 calorie diet			

Cucumber Mint Smoothie

Instead of sugar, this light and creamy drink has a tang of lemon and the pizzazz of mint to complement the creamy base.

1 cup peeled, seeded, and chopped cucumber
1 cup yogurt
1 cup milk
¼ teaspoon lemon juice
¼ cup chopped mint

Serves 2

The cucumber provides electrolytes, while the milk and yogurt give this combo protein and a creamy base. The formula is excellent for those with hypoglycemia, as it is extremely low in sugar and high in protein.

SERVING SIZE: ½ OF RECIPE (306G)			
CALORIES: 150		**CALORIES FROM FAT: 35**	
	%DV*		%DV*
Total Fat 4g	6%	Sugars 15g	
Saturated Fat 2.5g	13%	Protein 12g	
Cholesterol 15mg	5%	Vitamin A	15%
Sodium 160mg	7%	Vitamin C	6%
Total Carbohydrate 17g	6%	Calcium	35%
Dietary Fiber 1g	4%	Iron	2%
*Percent Daily Values are based on a 2,000 calorie diet			

Blueberry Crème Freeze

Blueberry heaven and nothing less. A rich decadent blend that goes easy on the calories and sugar.

1 cup ice cubes
1 cup milk
1 cup frozen blueberries
¼ cup cottage cheese
1 tablespoon toasted wheat germ
1 teaspoon xylitol
Optional: ¼ teaspoon vanilla extract

Serves 2

Blueberries do not raise blood sugar levels and are therefore an excellent fruit choice for those with diabetes. Xylitol is also a safe sweetener for diabetics.

SERVING SIZE: ½ OF RECIPE (350G)			
CALORIES: 150		**CALORIES FROM FAT: 50**	
	%DV*		%DV*
Total Fat 6g	9%	Sugars 14g	
Saturated Fat 3g	15%	Protein 9g	
Cholesterol 15mg	5%	Vitamin A	4%
Sodium 150mg	6%	Vitamin C	4%
Total Carbohydrate 18g	6%	Calcium	15%
Dietary Fiber 3g	12%	Iron	2%
*Percent Daily Values are based on a 2,000 calorie diet			

Strawberry Lemonade

Mint leaves, as a garnish, look beautiful against this creamy pink drink.

2 cups ice cubes
1 cup strawberry juice
½ cup lemon juice
¼ cup nonfat dry milk powder
Optional: mint leaves for garnish

Serves 2

Strawberries contain soluble fiber that helps slow the absorption of their natural sugars, therefore they do not raise blood sugar levels the way other fruit juices might. This smoothie also offers protein from the nonfat dry milk.

SERVING SIZE: ½ OF RECIPE (395G)			
CALORIES: 70		**CALORIES FROM FAT: 5**	
	%DV*		%DV*
Total Fat 0g	0%	Sugars 13g	
Saturated Fat 0g	0%	Protein 4g	
Cholesterol 0mg	0%	Vitamin A	4%
Sodium 60mg	3%	Vitamin C	80%
Total Carbohydrate 15g	5%	Calcium	15%
Dietary Fiber 0g	0%	Iron	2%
*Percent Daily Values are based on a 2,000 calorie diet			

Apricots and Cream

This is a sweet and creamy whip that is rich in flavor from the nectar.

1 cup ice cubes
½ cup milk
½ cup pitted apricots
½ cup apricot nectar
½ cup cottage cheese
1 teaspoon wheat germ

Serves 2

Apricots are high in beta-carotene and low on the glycemic list. They offer the added benefits of potassium, fiber, and iron. Cottage cheese is an excellent source of protein.

SERVING SIZE: ½ OF RECIPE (339G)			
CALORIES: 150		CALORIES FROM FAT: 40	
	%DV*		%DV*
Total Fat 4.5g	7%	Sugars 17g	
Saturated Fat 2.5g	13%	Protein 10g	
Cholesterol 15mg	5%	Vitamin A	35%
Sodium 230mg	10%	Vitamin C	8%
Total Carbohydrate 19g	6%	Calcium	15%
Dietary Fiber 1g	4%	Iron	2%
*Percent Daily Values are based on a 2,000 calorie diet			

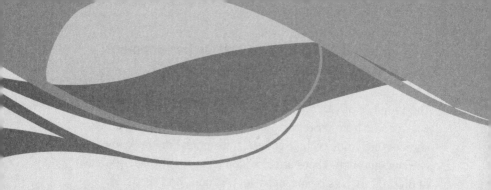

...Muscle Builders...

There are many benefits to gaining muscle mass, including more strength, control, and endurance. Recent research has confirmed that muscle development also leads to stronger bones and less risk for bone loss later in life.

By storing glycogen—the sugar that we use for endurance activities and to feed our brains—our muscles give us the camel-like ability to carry stored energy 24/7. To create the glycogen, we must take in calories. Accordingly, the more muscle we have, the more calories we need. In fact, for each pound of muscle we gain, authorities believe we burn an additional 100 to 150 calories in a twenty-four hour period. This is exciting news! What this means is that the more muscle we gain, the more calories that go into building and maintaining muscle mass, rather than becoming body fat. The math is fun for this equation. For example, if you gain 10 pounds of muscle, you are burning between 1,000 and 1,500 more calories in just one day. That's one of the reasons body builders have to eat such huge amounts of food.

By infusing your body with nutrients daily, you can provide your body with the elements it needs to build muscle efficiently as you work out.

Nutritional Guidelines for Muscle Development

Protein

The building blocks for muscle development are amino acids, which come from protein foods. Animal foods are good protein sources, including cottage cheese, milk, nonfat dry milk powder, chicken, and fish. There are also some excellent plant sources of protein, such as beans, peas, lentils, nuts, and seeds.

Essential Fatty Acids

Essential fatty acids (EFAs) are key for proper muscle development. There are several forms that are essential to your diet, as the body can't naturally make them. These include plant oils from foods such as avocado, nuts, and seeds, and omega-3 oils, which come from animal foods such as fish.

Minerals

Minerals are needed for cells to divide and grow into muscles. These include iron, zinc, sodium, potassium, magnesium, chromium, and manganese.

Bioflavonoids

Bioflavonoids such as hesperetin, hesperidin, eriodictyol, quercetin, and rutin are used extensively to treat athletic injuries because they relieve pain, bumps, and bruises. Bioflavonoids act synergistically with vitamin C to protect and preserve the structure of capillary blood vessels.

Lecithin

Studies show that lecithin, which contains choline, improves performance and reduces fatigue for runners, triathletes, basketball players, and swimmers. In one of the first studies in this area, researchers found that the blood choline levels of Boston

Marathon runners dropped by about 40 percent during the race. Choline supplementation prior to activity appears to prevent the decline of plasma choline and, in many cases, to improve performance.

Electrolytes

Calcium, magnesium, sodium, potassium, and chloride are known collectively as electrolytes. They are necessary for proper muscle movement—calcium for contraction and magnesium for relaxation. To build muscle, the fibers need to be able to relax fully and contract fully. Electrolytes are also important for performance, endurance, and the fatigue reduction associated with proper hydration. Magnesium is a muscle-relaxing mineral found in nuts, seeds, and chocolate. Calcium is needed not only for muscle contraction but also for bone formation. It is found in dairy foods, nuts, seeds, and soy products.

Athlete's Edge

This slushy tastes like grape pop, but it's loaded with nutrients an athlete needs!

¼ cup frozen grape juice concentrate
1 cup ice cubes
2 tablespoons nonfat dry milk powder
½ teaspoon electrolyte powder
1 teaspoon orange-flavored fish oil
Optional: ¼ teaspoon vitamin C

Serves 1

The juice provides glucose for energy, so that your body can be refueled. The milk powder is a source of protein, and the ice, electrolytes, and fish oil help hydrate the muscles.

SERVING SIZE: 1 (324G)			
CALORIES: 200		**CALORIES FROM FAT: 45**	
	%DV*		%DV*
Total Fat 5g	8%	Sugars 36g	
Saturated Fat 1g	5%	Protein 3g	
Cholesterol 25mg	8%	Vitamin A	90%
Sodium 60mg	3%	Vitamin C	100%
Total Carbohydrate 36g	12%	Calcium	20%
Dietary Fiber 0g	0%	Iron	2%
*Percent Daily Values are based on a 2,000 calorie diet			

Ginger Peach

This thick and juicy sorbet has a spicy edge that's not to be missed.

1 cup peach nectar
½ cup frozen peach slices
¼ cup cottage cheese
1 teaspoon honey
⅛ teaspoon ground ginger

Serves 1

Peaches are a concentrated source of muscle-protecting carotenoids. The cottage cheese provides about 8 grams of protein, and the ginger warms the digestive tract, which stimulates digestion and the absorption of nutrients.

SERVING SIZE: 1 (383G)			
CALORIES: 240		**CALORIES FROM FAT: 20**	
	%DV*		%DV*
Total Fat 2.5g	4%	Sugars 47g	
Saturated Fat 1.5g	8%	Protein 8g	
Cholesterol 10mg	3%	Vitamin A	20%
Sodium 220mg	9%	Vitamin C	140%
Total Carbohydrate 49g	16%	Calcium	6%
Dietary Fiber 2g	8%	Iron	4%
*Percent Daily Values are based on a 2,000 calorie diet			

Chocolate Pudding Shake

This delicious snack is loaded with muscle-building compounds.

½ cup ice cubes
½ cup milk
½ cup silken tofu
½ cup unsweetened cocoa powder
1 frozen peeled banana
3 tablespoons nonfat dry milk powder
Optional: ¼ teaspoon vanilla extract

Serves 2

Cocoa is a potent source of antioxidants that protect tissue and boost the immune system, while the banana is full of potassium, which helps facilitate muscle movement. The milk and tofu provide protein.

SERVING SIZE: ½ OF RECIPE (263G)			
CALORIES: 210		**CALORIES FROM FAT: 50**	
	%DV*		%DV*
Total Fat 6g	9%	Sugars 13g	
Saturated Fat 1g	5%	Protein 13g	
Cholesterol 5mg	2%	Vitamin A	4%
Sodium 90mg	4%	Vitamin C	10%
Total Carbohydrate 33g	11%	Calcium	15%
Dietary Fiber 6g	24%	Iron	10%
*Percent Daily Values are based on a 2,000 calorie diet			

Coconut Frosty

This tropical delight is a creamy and decadent blend of healthy ingredients.

1 cup ice cubes
½ cup milk
¼ cup nonfat dry milk or protein powder
½ cup crushed pineapple
½ cup ice cream
2 tablespoons coconut oil

Serves 2

When you need a protein hit and really want to treat yourself, this protein-packed combination has more than enough carbohydrates to last through a tough workout.

SERVING SIZE: ½ OF RECIPE (281G)			
CALORIES: 290		**CALORIES FROM FAT: 170**	
	%DV*		%DV*
Total Fat 20g	31%	Sugars 17g	
Saturated Fat 15g	75%	Protein 11g	
Cholesterol 35mg	12%	Vitamin A	4%
Sodium 75mg	3%	Vitamin C	8%
Total Carbohydrate 18g	6%	Calcium	20%
Dietary Fiber 1g	4%	Iron	2%
*Percent Daily Values are based on a 2,000 calorie diet			

Banana Bread Smoothie

There's nothing quite so tempting as warm banana bread, but this smoothie comes close, with its rich mix of walnuts, milk, and frozen bananas.

¼ cup walnuts
1 frozen peeled banana
1 cup milk
¼ cup wheat germ
¼ teaspoon grated nutmeg

Serves 2

Walnuts contain essential fatty acids that reduce inflammation; bananas provide the mineral potassium; and the milk is a good source of protein. Toasted wheat germ contains Coenzyme Q_{10} (CoQ10), which can restore the enzymatic action in fat cells, which allows the release of stored fat. Toasted wheat germ is the perfect CoQ10-containing food to add to smoothies as it blends well, has very little taste, and almost disappears in a creamy drink.

SERVING SIZE: ½ OF RECIPE (211G)			
CALORIES: 280		**CALORIES FROM FAT: 140**	
	%DV*		%DV*
Total Fat 15g	23%	Sugars 16g	
Saturated Fat 3.5g	18%	Protein 11g	
Cholesterol 10mg	3%	Vitamin A	4%
Sodium 50mg	2%	Vitamin C	8%
Total Carbohydrate 28g	9%	Calcium	15%
Dietary Fiber 6g	24%	Iron	10%
*Percent Daily Values are based on a 2,000 calorie diet			

Malted Frapoothie

Like an old-fashioned malted milkshake, but a whole lot healthier!

½ cup ice cream
½ cup ice cubes
½ cup milk
¼ cup protein powder
1 tablespoon unsweetened cocoa powder
1 tablespoon malted milk powder
¼ teaspoon electrolyte powder
Optional: 2 teaspoons instant coffee crystals

Serves 2

This creamy shake is rich in protein from the dairy products and protein powder and contains malt, a good source of B vitamins. The antioxidants in the cocoa protect muscles from the oxidizing effects of stress-related hormones such as cortisol, which can develop as a reaction to very strenuous exercise.

SERVING SIZE: ½ OF RECIPE (177G)			
CALORIES: 200		**CALORIES FROM FAT: 70**	
	%DV*		%DV*
Total Fat 7g	11%	Sugars 15g	
Saturated Fat 4g	20%	Protein 13g	
Cholesterol 40mg	13%	Vitamin A	4%
Sodium 115mg	5%	Vitamin C	0%
Total Carbohydrate 20g	7%	Calcium	25%
Dietary Fiber 1g	4%	Iron	2%
*Percent Daily Values are based on a 2,000 calorie diet			

Papaya Lime

Papaya is a largely underestimated fruit. This creamy tropical shake is loaded with high-quality, muscle-building nutrients.

1 papaya, seeded and peeled
½ cup papaya nectar
½ cup ice cubes
1 tablespoon lime juice
1 teaspoon honey
2 tablespoons protein powder or cottage cheese

Serves 1

Papaya is full of carotenoids, which protect cells from the sun's ultraviolet rays and from environmental toxins. Body-building involves the formation of new cells, which need to be protected as they divide and grow. Beta-carotene and a full range of carotenoids are protective of cells and support immune function.

SERVING SIZE: 1 (416G)			
CALORIES: 190		**CALORIES FROM FAT: 10**	
	%DV*		%DV*
Total Fat 1g	2%	Sugars 32g	
Saturated Fat 0g	1%	Protein 9g	
Cholesterol 15mg	5%	Vitamin A	40%
Sodium 35mg	1%	Vitamin C	160%
Total Carbohydrate 39g	13%	Calcium	15%
Dietary Fiber 3g	12%	Iron	4%
*Percent Daily Values are based on a 2,000 calorie diet			

Strawberry Shake

The heady sweetness of a vanilla bean gives this shake an exotic twist.

1 cup milk
1 cup ice cream
2 cups strawberries
1 scoop vanilla protein powder or
⅓ cup nonfat dry milk powder
Optional: 1 teaspoon minced vanilla bean
1 teaspoon barley malt

Serves 2

Nonfat dry milk powder is an inexpensive and easy way to add protein to drinks. Just ⅓ cup contains 8 grams of protein and dissolves well in smoothies.

SERVING SIZE: ½ OF RECIPE (427G)			
CALORIES: 330		**CALORIES FROM FAT: 110**	
	%DV*		%DV*
Total Fat 13g	20%	Sugars 33g	
Saturated Fat 7g	35%	Protein 16g	
Cholesterol 60mg	20%	Vitamin A	8%
Sodium 125mg	5%	Vitamin C	220%
Total Carbohydrate 42g	14%	Calcium	30%
Dietary Fiber 5g	20%	Iron	6%
*Percent Daily Values are based on a 2,000 calorie diet			

Mocha Frapoothie

Peanut butter has made its name in the health world for good reason. Here, the PB is barely overpowered by milk and yummy cocoa for a thick energy-filled drink.

1 cup ice cubes
1 cup milk
½ cup peanut butter
¼ cup unsweetened cocoa powder
1 tablespoon nutritional yeast

Serves 2

Nutritional yeast is an excellent source of B vitamins and blends well in smoothies. The B vitamins, such as B_2, B_3, B_{12}, and pantothenic acid, are necessary for energy production and for turning calories into muscle.

SERVING SIZE: ½ OF RECIPE (316G)			
CALORIES: 490		**CALORIES FROM FAT: 330**	
	%DV*		%DV*
Total Fat 37g	57%	Sugars 11g	
Saturated Fat 7g	35%	Protein 22g	
Cholesterol 10mg	3%	Vitamin A	2%
Sodium 360mg	15%	Vitamin C	0%
Total Carbohydrate 26g	9%	Calcium	15%
Dietary Fiber 7g	28%	Iron	10%
*Percent Daily Values are based on a 2,000 calorie diet			

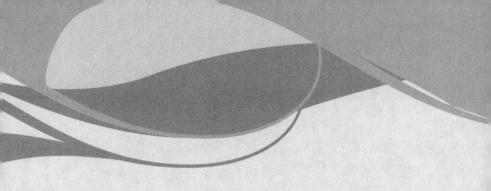

...Libido...

A healthy sex drive and adequate sexual response are hall-marks of general well-being. Everyone has his or her own ideas about how active the libido should be. Lucky are the partners whose appetites are in synch, yet rarely do those appetites stay constant. Some problem concerning intimacy happens to nearly every adult in a relationship eventually, but the worst thing we can do in this situation is to take offense, assign blame, or assume that there is a deeper problem without checking in with each other. Assuming there is good communication and any underlying emotional conflicts that may be preventing intimacy have been addressed, the next step is to look at nutritional strategies for keeping the spark of passion alight.

General Nutrition Guidelines

Avoid Hydrogenated and Saturated Fats

Unhealthy oils, such as saturated fats, trans fats, and hydrogenated oil, raise cholesterol in the blood, which can harden in the arteries and restrict blood flow. This is counter to a healthy sexual response, which involves dilated blood vessels to rush nutrients and hormones through the body via the vascular system. Furthermore, high heat used in cooking these fats changes their chemical structure and creates toxins that interfere with formation of sex hormones. Use only fresh oils and avoid eating too many processed foods.

Reduce Refined Carbohydrates

Sugars feed the brain, muscles, fatty tissue, and sex organs; the surplus can be stored in muscles and liver as glycogen, or potential fuel. Good sugar, in healthy doses, is necessary, but in too many of the foods we eat we overdo the sugar. By skipping simple sugars and refined carbohydrates such as those in soft drinks, alcohol, white bread, white flour products, and most pastas, you can do wonders for your health and put your body back in balance. These foods are depleted of vitamins and minerals and must borrow from our bodily stores, which leads to nutrient deficiencies that can seriously reduce amorous activities.

Eat Complex Carbohydrates

Complex carbohydrates such as vegetables, fruits, beans, nuts, seeds, and whole grains contain vitamins, minerals, fiber, and other nutrients that are necessary for heightened energy and healthy blood flow. Fiber (soluble and insoluble), such as the pectin in fruit, and cellulose help slow the absorption of nutrients, making for a greater endurance, and they also detoxify the system and reduce cholesterol.

Libido-Enhancing Ingredients

Chiles (Capsaicin)

Vanillin is in the class of vanilloids, which includes the hot spice capsaicin, found in chiles. The vanilloid receptors of the central and peripheral nervous systems bind with this compound, resulting in heightened sensory effects. Chiles, like citrus fruits, contain concentrated amounts of vitamin C. Lack of this important vitamin can result in infertility and reduction of drive.

Chocolate

Chocolate contains the amino acid arginine, which directly increases sperm production. Chocolate and cocoa also contain a natural chemical called theobromine, a stimulant frequently confused with caffeine. In fact, theobromine has very different effects on the human body from caffeine; it is a mild, longer-lasting stimulant with a strong mood-improving effect.

Dark chocolate and cocoa contain three substances from the chemical group N-acylethanolamine. These substances stimulate the area of the brain that produces feelings of pleasure and are similar to the chemicals found in marijuana. One of these substances, phenylethylalamine, is found in increased quantities in our bodies when we are in love and during the sexual act. During metabolism, chocolate breaks down into amino acids, which also directly affect the production of the "feel good" neurotransmitter serotonin.

Cinnamon

Cinnamon and cloves both increase the effectiveness of the hormone insulin, which allows your body to use glucose for energy even more efficiently. Cinnamon has been touted as an aphrodisiac for centuries.

Cloves

Cloves are the dried flower buds of *Jambosa caryophyllus*, also called *Eugenia caryophyllata* and *Caryophyllus aromaticus*. Cloves were considered an aphrodisiac in Asia and China as early as the third century B.C. The main constituent of cloves and clove oil is eugenol, but small quantities of furfural, vanillin, and methyl amyl ketone are also present. Eugenol from cloves is a mild anesthesia and was once a dental analgesic.

Flavored Fish Oil

Eicosapentaenoic acid (EPA) is an omega-3 fatty acid and is the only known source (other than mother's milk) of both linoleic acid (LA) and gamma-linolenic acid (GLA). They are both necessary for the production of prostaglandins, which regulate a wide range of body functions including blood pressure, cholesterol levels, and sexual hormone response. GLA is found in borage oil, hemp, primrose, and flaxseed oil.

A deficiency in EPA leads to a number of dysfunctions, including the disruption of cellular response to sexual stimuli. EPA deficiency also leads to increased menstrual cramping and increased incidence of infertility. Fish oil also contains vitamin B_6, which helps convert linoleic acid into prostaglandins. It is found in fish oils of cod liver, herring, mackerel, salmon, and sardine. Flavored fish oils such as the orange-flavored Coromega and liquid Udòs Oil taste great in smoothies.

Flaxseed

Flaxseed contain essential fatty acids (EFAs), the building blocks of the hormone-like substances called prostaglandins, which are necessary for sexual response. Dietary support for prostaglandin production is an effective treatment for impotency for many men. Flaxseed provides soluble and insoluble fibers that aid in reducing and maintaining proper cholesterol levels. Daily intake of flaxseed also enhances vascular dilation.

Ginger

Ginger consists of the dried rhizomes of *Zingiber officinale* (Zingiberaceae). The active compounds are called gingerols, and they have medicinal properties that promote circulation and increase the dilation of blood vessels, an integral part of sexual function.

Lecithin

Lecithin contains choline (acetylcholine), which is the primary chemical the body uses to transmit signals from nerves to skeletal muscles. There is reason to believe that enhancing cholinergic neurotransmuscular transmission will enhance your energy and stamina.

Phosphorus combines with nitrogen, fatty acids, and glycerol to form phospholipids, including lecithin, which helps promote the secretion of glandular hormones and sex hormones. Lecithin can be added to the diet to assist in correcting muscle weakness, glandular exhaustion, and nerve disorders.

Licorice Root

Licorice root comes from the European leguminous plant *Glycyrrhiza glabra* and has been shown to affect estrogen levels and work as a phytoestrogen. This natural plant estrogen is helpful in balancing female hormones, which supports libido.

Nutritional Yeast

Women on the contraceptive pill often have diminished serum levels of folic acid and vitamin B_6, which can both be replenished via nutritional yeast. There have been suggestions that such vitamin supplementation may help overcome depression and diminished libido in some women on the pill.

Nuts and Seeds

Nuts and seeds contain vitamin E, which affects male sex hormone production. Vitamin E is found in concentrations in the anterior pituitary gland, where it protects sexual hormones such as testosterone from oxidation, keeping them working in the bloodstream longer. Deficiency of vitamin E can lead to deterioration of the reproductive system. This nutrient has also been used to relieve PMS symptoms, such as backache and muscular discomfort, and menopause symptoms such as hot flashes.

Soybeans

Soybeans contain several amino acids that play specific roles in the physiology of sexual response. Soybeans provide phenylalanine, tryptophan, and tyrosine, which are precursors to many of the sexual arousal and response neurotransmitters. Our bodies use these amino acids to make the chemicals that regulate our mood, including serotonin, dopamine, and norepinephrine.

Dietary intake of soy will often reverse deficiency-related depression and lack of sexual drive. Soybeans also contain tryptophan, an amino acid necessary for the production of serotonin in the brain. Tryptophan plays an important role in the physiology of an orgasm by inducing vasoconstriction and contraction. The one hormonal caveat with soy products is they interfere with thyroid activity, so if you are taking synthroid or have experienced hypothyroidism, you should try to avoid soy.

Tea

Tea leaves (*Camellia thea*) contain the chemical theophylline, which dilates the coronary artery carrying blood to the heart and throughout the body.

Vanilla

Vanilla is a well-known powerful aphrodisiac, acting through its scent as much as through its taste. Vanilla is the cured, full-grown, unripe fruit of an orchid, *Vanilla planifolia*. It derives from the Spanish word *vainila*, a diminutive of *vaina*, meaning "pod." Vanilla must be taken in larger amounts than most food products to obtain noticeable effects; however, it has been shown to have a stimulating effect on the motor nerves used in sexual response. Participants who consumed the vanilla from one to two vanilla beans experienced some sexual stimulation.

It is important to use real vanilla rather than synthetic vanillin, which is cheaper but less effective. Real vanilla extract or vanilla beans can be found in most natural food stores.

Vitamin E

Vitamin E supports the integrity of red blood cells that carry oxygen and iron through the bloodstream to the sexual organs. It is necessary for the health of the testes, hormone production (specifically progesterone), and function of the pituitary gland, which has profound control over the sexual organs, sexual characteristics, and sexual function in both males and females. Aim for 600 international units of natural mixed tocopherols daily. These can be found in wheat germ oil, sunflower seeds, sunflower oil, almonds, sesame seeds, olive oil, and soybean oil. Peanuts are a rich source of vitamin E.

Wheat Germ and Wheat Bran

Essential fatty acids from unhydrogenated oils such as those found in wheat germ actually lower cholesterol levels and reverse the negative effects of bad oils. Sex research by the physician members of the Academy of Orthomolecular Psychiatry indicated that certain types of dietary fiber—such as wheat bran, whole apples, the pulp from citrus foods, and the red skins of peanut seeds—help maintain the integrity of the body organs involved with sexuality, such as the liver, adrenals, and pancreas.

Zinc

Zinc is necessary for fertility and sexual drive. Zinc deficiency can cause sexual dysfunction, reduced sperm production, lowered semen output, reduced testosterone levels, and reduced energy. Zinc is so important for hormone production that pre-pubescent individuals experience delayed sexual maturity when deficient in this important mineral. Pumpkin seeds, pumpkin seed butter, toasted wheat germ, and dairy foods are all good sources of zinc.

Mauna Kea Mango

Mango nectar is a miracle ingredient for smoothies. Nectar is a pulpy juice that adds tremendous flavor and depth to blender drinks.

1 cup ice cubes
1 cup mango nectar
½ cup strawberries
½ papaya, peeled and seeded
Optional: 1 mango (about 1 cup), peeled and pitted

Serves 2

Fruit contains natural sugars and electrolytes that boost energy and stimulate blood flow.

SERVING SIZE: ½ OF RECIPE (336G)			
CALORIES: 100		**CALORIES FROM FAT: 5**	
	%DV*		%DV*
Total Fat 0g	0%	Sugars 20g	
Saturated Fat 0g	0%	Protein 1g	
Cholesterol 0mg	0%	Vitamin A	25%
Sodium 15mg	1%	Vitamin C	120%
Total Carbohydrate 24g	8%	Calcium	4%
Dietary Fiber 2g	8%	Iron	4%
*Percent Daily Values are based on a 2,000 calorie diet			

Coconut Blueberry Shake

This interesting blueberry shake is creamy and slightly sweet, with a hint of warming ginger and tropical coconut.

2 cups nonfat milk
2 cups frozen blueberries
1 teaspoon flaxseed oil
6 tablespoons protein powder
1 tablespoon wheat germ
1 teaspoon ground ginger
1 tablespoon shredded dried coconut

Serves 4

The antioxidants from blueberries assist in the burning of body fat for energy, and the vasodilating effects of ginger and the essential fatty acids from the flaxseed oil help blood move throughout the body, thus supporting sexual function.

SERVING SIZE: ¼ OF RECIPE (214G)			
CALORIES: 140		**CALORIES FROM FAT: 25**	
	%DV*		%DV*
Total Fat 2.5g	4%	Sugars 14g	
Saturated Fat 0.5g	3%	Protein 11g	
Cholesterol 15mg	5%	Vitamin A	6%
Sodium 85mg	4%	Vitamin C	4%
Total Carbohydrate 18g	6%	Calcium	20%
Dietary Fiber 3g	12%	Iron	2%
*Percent Daily Values are based on a 2,000 calorie diet			

Pure Joy

Nutmeg and cinnamon really bring out the flavor of the cantaloupe in this sweet and spicy icy.

2 cups cantaloupe
1 cup ice cubes
¼ teaspoon grated nutmeg
½ teaspoon ground cinnamon

Serves 2

The compound responsible for the allegedly hallucinogenic and possibly aphrodisiacal effects of nutmeg is myristicin, which has some structural similarity with mescaline, the hallucinogen from the peyote cactus.

SERVING SIZE: ½ OF RECIPE (279G)			
CALORIES: 60		**CALORIES FROM FAT: 5**	
	%DV*		%DV*
Total Fat 0g	0%	Sugars 12g	
Saturated Fat 0g	0%	Protein 1g	
Cholesterol 0mg	0%	Vitamin A	110%
Sodium 30mg	1%	Vitamin C	100%
Total Carbohydrate 14g	5%	Calcium	2%
Dietary Fiber 2g	8%	Iron	4%
*Percent Daily Values are based on a 2,000 calorie diet			

Good and Plenty

Just like the candy, but cold and creamy! This one is for girls only. Read on to find out why.

1 cup milk
1 cup vanilla yogurt
½ cup ice cubes
1 teaspoon licorice extract

Serves 2

Vanilla is a natural aphrodisiac, as is licorice root, which contains phytoestrogens that support female libido. Unfortunately, these same phytoestrogens compete with testosterone, so this one is not recommended for men.

SERVING SIZE: ½ OF RECIPE (298G)			
CALORIES: 150		**CALORIES FROM FAT: 50**	
	%DV*		%DV*
Total Fat 5g	8%	Sugars 16g	
Saturated Fat 3.5g	18%	Protein 9g	
Cholesterol 20mg	7%	Vitamin A	6%
Sodium 130mg	5%	Vitamin C	2%
Total Carbohydrate 16g	5%	Calcium	30%
Dietary Fiber 0g	0%	Iron	0%
*Percent Daily Values are based on a 2,000 calorie diet			

Exceptional-E Male

Now here's a good one for the fellas.

1 cup milk
1 frozen peeled banana
¼ cup peanut butter or almond butter
2 tablespoons toasted wheat germ

Serves 2

Studies show that vitamin E keeps the sex hormone testosterone from breaking down in the bloodstream as quickly, therefore sustaining its libido-driving effects over a longer period of time. Nuts and nut butter contain significant amounts of vitamin E.

SERVING SIZE: ½ OF RECIPE (221G)			
CALORIES: 340		**CALORIES FROM FAT: 190**	
	%DV*		%DV*
Total Fat 21g	32%	Sugars 17g	
Saturated Fat 5g	25%	Protein 14g	
Cholesterol 10mg	3%	Vitamin A	4%
Sodium 210mg	9%	Vitamin C	8%
Total Carbohydrate 29g	10%	Calcium	15%
Dietary Fiber 6g	24%	Iron	8%
*Percent Daily Values are based on a 2,000 calorie diet			

Mexican Chocolate Smoothie

My favorite cocoa is made by Dagoba. In this spicy shake, I use their organic cocoa called Xocolatl, with chiles and cinnamon. It's delicious!

1 cup milk
½ cup ice cubes
½ cup cottage cheese
3 tablespoons unsweetened cocoa powder
¼ teaspoon chili powder
¼ teaspoon ground cinnamon

Serves 1

Here the natural oils in the chile powder stimulate the peripheral nervous systems, the chocolate increases the production of the neurotransmitter serotonin (the pleasure hormone), and the cinnamon helps the body break down calories from the dairy products for lasting energy.

SERVING SIZE: 1 (493G)			
CALORIES: 290		**CALORIES FROM FAT: 130**	
	%DV*		%DV*
Total Fat 14g	22%	Sugars 15g	
Saturated Fat 8g	40%	Protein 24g	
Cholesterol 40mg	13%	Vitamin A	15%
Sodium 510mg	21%	Vitamin C	0%
Total Carbohydrate 25g	8%	Calcium	40%
Dietary Fiber 4g	16%	Iron	8%
*Percent Daily Values are based on a 2,000 calorie diet			

Vanilla Dreamsicle

Orange juice, banana, and vanilla combine to create a remarkable simulation of a favorite yesteryear treat.

1 cup orange juice
1 frozen peeled banana
1 tablespoon lecithin granules or liquid
1 teaspoon nutritional yeast
1 teaspoon minced vanilla bean

Serves 1

Nutritional yeast boosts B vitamin levels, which can improve mood, while the vanilla serves as a potent aphrodisiac.

SERVING SIZE: 1 (375G)			
CALORIES: 280		**CALORIES FROM FAT: 45**	
	%DV*		%DV*
Total Fat 5g	8%	Sugars 35g	
Saturated Fat 1g	5%	Protein 4g	
Cholesterol 0mg	0%	Vitamin A	10%
Sodium 0mg	0%	Vitamin C	220%
Total Carbohydrate 54g	18%	Calcium	6%
Dietary Fiber 4g	16%	Iron	6%
*Percent Daily Values are based on a 2,000 calorie diet			

Chocolate Seduction

Light on calories but rich in flavor, this whip has secret "libido-enhancing" nutrients in its seductive chocolate-almond base.

1 cup almond milk
1 cup ice cubes
4 tablespoons unsweetened cocoa powder
1 tablespoon nutritional yeast
1 teaspoon minced vanilla bean

Serves 2

Vanilla directly stimulates nerves, often producing a heightened sense of touch; the nutritional yeast provides B vitamins, which support energy production and nerve growth; and the cocoa provides the phytochemicals needed by the cells in the brain and digestive tract to produce the sensual neurotransmitters.

SERVING SIZE: ½ OF RECIPE (251G)			
CALORIES: 70		**CALORIES FROM FAT: 25**	
	%DV*		%DV*
Total Fat 2.5g	4%	Sugars 4g	
Saturated Fat 0g	0%	Protein 3g	
Cholesterol 0mg	0%	Vitamin A	6%
Sodium 80mg	3%	Vitamin C	0%
Total Carbohydrate 11g	4%	Calcium	10%
Dietary Fiber 3g	12%	Iron	6%
*Percent Daily Values are based on a 2,000 calorie diet			

Love Elixir

Exotic and spicy, this *Kama Sutra*–inspired shake combines the flavors and scents of India.

1 cup milk
1 cup plain yogurt
½ cup ice cubes
2 tablespoons tahini
3 dates, pitted
⅛ teaspoon ground cardamom
⅛ teaspoon ground cinnamon
1 teaspoon minced vanilla bean

Serves 2

Tahini is a sesame seed paste that naturally contains calcium and B vitamins. Calcium is the mineral necessary for orgasmic muscle contractions. Vitamin B_3 (niacin) dilates the blood vessels and increases the blood flow necessary for the physical and biochemical demands of sexual activity.

SERVING SIZE: ½ OF RECIPE (347G)			
CALORIES: 330		**CALORIES FROM FAT: 120**	
	%DV*		%DV*
Total Fat 13g	20%	Sugars 39g	
Saturated Fat 3.5g	18%	Protein 16g	
Cholesterol 15mg	5%	Vitamin A	15%
Sodium 170mg	7%	Vitamin C	0%
Total Carbohydrate 43g	14%	Calcium	40%
Dietary Fiber 3g	12%	Iron	10%
*Percent Daily Values are based on a 2,000 calorie diet			

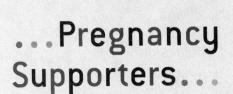

...Pregnancy Supporters...

Pregnancy can be one of the most nutritionally demanding stages in a woman's life, as gestation involves rapid cell division and organ development for both the mother and the fetus. A weight gain of 25 to 35 pounds is considered normal for a healthy woman. This requires an extra 300 calories a day from nutritionally dense foods that need to supply specific macro- and micro-nutrients to the fetus and the mother's body.

General Nutrition Guidelines

Protein

Pregnancy increases the need for protein by about 10 grams per day in the first trimester and by 21 grams per day in the second and third trimesters. Adding protein-rich foods to smoothies, such as cottage cheese, which has a whopping 13 grams of protein in just ½ cup; nut butter, such as peanut butter, hazelnut butter, and almond butter; nonfat dry milk powder; or protein powders is a tasty way to fulfill this requirement daily.

Folic Acid

Since mammals cannot synthesize (make) folic acid, we must take it in through our diet or through the by-products of intestinal organisms (microflora). Folic acid is essential for the biosynthesis of amino acids, neurotransmitters, purines, and pyramidines, hence DNA and RNA, and is also necessary for cell division as the fetus develops and grows. Doctors recommend 400 to 600 mcg per day. Folate is the general term for this nutrient; folic acid is the synthetic form used in supplements and in fortified grain products. Taking folic acid before and during early pregnancy can reduce the risk of spina bifida and other neural tube defects in infants. Good sources of folate are citrus fruits and juices, peanuts, and whole grains.

Essential Fatty Acids

Pregnant women have a high requirement for lipid-soluble vitamins and essential fatty acids. Fish oils contain DHA (docosahexaenoic acid) and EPA (eicosapentaenoic acid), which play a role in the brain development and visual function of developing infants. Gamma-linolenic acid (GLA) is an omega-6 fatty acid found in borage oil, primrose, and hemp. It is necessary for supporting prostaglandin production and reducing inflammation. These and other flavored fish oils can be added to almost any smoothie.

Taurine

Babies get the essential amino acid taurine through breast milk. Mothers get it by eating methionine-rich foods such as cottage cheese, peanuts, cashews, and pistachios, which our livers then convert to taurine before it is passed on to the baby to assist in cell development and growth.

Calcium

Studies have indicated that calcium supplements may reduce the risk of preclampsia and hypertension in pregnant women. Calcium may also reduce the risk of pregnancy complications, according to a study in the *American Journal of Obstetrics and Gynecology.*

A new study found that when a group of pregnant women were given 1,500 mg of calcium a day (the recommended dose is 1,000 mg), they had 25 percent fewer complications, such as kidney problems, headaches, and changes in vision from severe preclampsia, a disorder that causes very high blood pressure, than a counterpart group that took a placebo. Their babies were also less likely to die in their first four weeks of life. Taking 1,500 mg of calcium a day is as simple as adding two servings of yogurt and two glasses of milk to your daily diet; 1,500 mg can also be obtained from a supplement, and daily from green foods such as broccoli, summer squash, and spinach.

Calcium-rich foods that make good smoothie ingredients are listed below in order from the greatest to the least amount of calcium per serving.

SERVING SIZE	FOOD	CALCIUM (mg)
1 cup	Plain yogurt, nonfat	452
1 cup	Plain yogurt, low-fat	415
1 cup	Yogurt, fruit	343
½ cup	Ricotta cheese, part skim	335
1 cup	Milk, nonfat	302
1 cup	Milk, low-fat (1%)	300
1 cup	Milk, low-fat (2%)	297
1 cup	Milk, whole	291
1 cup	Buttermilk	285
½ cup	Ricotta cheese, whole milk	254
¼ cup	Condensed milk, sweetened	217

Magnesium

Magnesium is useful for calming and relaxing pregnant women and their tired muscles. Magnesium is the atom responsible for the green color of chlorophyll, therefore green vegetables are a dependable source. Powdered magnesium supplements such as Natural Calm can also be added to smoothies.

Prebiotics

Prebiotic oligosaccharides such as inulin are now being added to yogurt and other probiotic-containing products. These support the growth of the probiotics, which are living microbial organisms necessary for gut health. There are hundreds of different organisms that colonize our digestive tract. Lactobacilli and bifidobacteria are two of the most well known because they are in yogurt, but broader range supplements containing freeze-dried cultures (in capsules or powder form) or in prepared fermented dairy products can also be added to smoothies. Probiotics are known for their ability to help ease diarrhea, yeast infections, food allergies, children's eczema, and even colds. Now research suggests another possible benefit: relieving intestinal disorders triggered by stress.

Choline

Choline is necessary for fetal and infant brain and mental development, and can be obtained through lecithin. Lecithin is abundant in our nerve cell membranes and is required for nerve growth and function, meaning it's very important for growing babies. Infant formulas approved by the FDA are required to contain levels of choline comparable to those in human milk. Lecithin can be purchased as dried granules or in liquid form.

Iron

The dietary need for iron doubles during pregnancy, and recommendations typically increase from 15 mg to 30 mg per day.

This additional iron is needed as a result of increased maternal blood volume. The fetus also stores enough iron to last through the first few months of life. Iron deficiency in the mother can lead to both low-birth-weight babies and a very tired mom. The following are food sources of iron.

SERVING SIZE	FOOD	IRON (mg)
2 tablespoons	Pumpkin seeds	8.6
3 ounces	Tofu, firm	8.5
2 tablespoons	Blackstrap molasses	6.4
3 ounces	Tofu, regular	6.2
2 tablespoons	Sunflower seeds	3.8
2 tablespoons	Cashews	3.4
2 tablespoons	Dried brewer's yeast	2.7
½ cup	Dandelion greens	2.3
2 tablespoons	Almonds	2.0
3 halves	Peaches, dried	1.9
½ cup	Raisins	1.5
3 dried	Figs	1.3
10 dried	Apricots	1.7

Blueberry Sparkler

This sweet bubbly is an excellent drink to have each day during pregnancy.

1 cup sparkling water
1 cup blueberry juice
1 cup ice cubes
10 drops liquid folic acid
¼ cup frozen apple juice concentrate

Serves 1

Liquid folic acid is so easy to add to smoothies, and it helps to reduce anxiety, depression, and prevent a folic acid deficiency in fetuses, which can result in spina bifida. Staying hydrated can also be a challenge during pregnancy, and this bubbly cocktail will replenish water and electrolytes to hydrate you and your baby.

SERVING SIZE: 1 (782G)			
CALORIES: 230		**CALORIES FROM FAT: 0**	
	%DV*		%DV*
Total Fat 0g	0%	Sugars 46g	
Saturated Fat 0g	0%	Protein 1g	
Cholesterol 0mg	0%	Vitamin A	0%
Sodium 70mg	3%	Vitamin C	2%
Total Carbohydrate 57g	19%	Calcium	10%
Dietary Fiber 0g	0%	Iron	8%
*Percent Daily Values are based on a 2,000 calorie diet			

Neuro Generator

This fruity blend is also appealing as a daily elixir.

½ cup mango juice
½ cup peach juice
½ cup ice cubes
¼ cup frozen apple juice concentrate
2 tablespoons orange-flavored fish oil (such as Coromega)
1 teaspoon nutritional yeast

Serves 2

This is nerve magic—the B vitamins from the nutritional yeast and the essential fatty acids from the fish oil are necessary for the baby's nerve growth and brain development.

SERVING SIZE: ½ OF RECIPE (255G)			
CALORIES: 280		**CALORIES FROM FAT: 120**	
	%DV*		%DV*
Total Fat 14g	22%	Sugars 38g	
Saturated Fat 3g	15%	Protein 1g	
Cholesterol 80mg	27%	Vitamin A	280%
Sodium 25mg	1%	Vitamin C	25%
Total Carbohydrate 40g	13%	Calcium	2%
Dietary Fiber 1g	2%	Iron	4%
*Percent Daily Values are based on a 2,000 calorie diet			

Pom Apple

Pomegranate juice tastes best with a bit of sweet juice. The rich apple flavor in the concentrate combines with the tart pomegranate to create a unique, flavorful taste experience.

½ cup pomegranate juice
½ cup sparkling water
½ cup apple juice concentrate
Optional: 1 teaspoon sweetener

Serves 1

Pomegranate and apple juice are rich sources of antioxidants that support the baby's development, as well as assisting the mother in fighting stress-related fatigue.

SERVING SIZE: 1 (358G)			
CALORIES: 260		**CALORIES FROM FAT: 5**	
	%DV*		%DV*
Total Fat 0g	0%	Sugars 61g	
Saturated Fat 0g	0%	Protein 1g	
Cholesterol 0mg	0%	Vitamin A	0%
Sodium 45mg	2%	Vitamin C	4%
Total Carbohydrate 64g	21%	Calcium	6%
Dietary Fiber 0g	0%	Iron	0%
*Percent Daily Values are based on a 2,000 calorie diet			

Stomach Soother

This delicate blend of soothing ingredients calms upset stomachs and minds.

½ cup yogurt
½ cup rice milk
1 banana, fresh or frozen, peeled
Optional: powdered microflora supplements

Serves 1

Yogurt contains microflora that aids digestion, rice milk is soothing (and the least allergenic of all milk options), and bananas provide protein and sooth sensitive stomachs and intestines.

SERVING SIZE: 1 (354G)			
CALORIES: 230		**CALORIES FROM FAT: 10**	
	%DV*		%DV*
Total Fat 1.5g	2%	Sugars 23g	
Saturated Fat 0g	0%	Protein 9g	
Cholesterol 5mg	2%	Vitamin A	10%
Sodium 160mg	7%	Vitamin C	20%
Total Carbohydrate 49g	16%	Calcium	20%
Dietary Fiber 3g	12%	Iron	2%
*Percent Daily Values are based on a 2,000 calorie diet			

Calcium Protection

Creamy, cool, and soothing, this milk chocolate mix makes for a sweet afternoon pick-me-up.

1 cup ice cubes
1 cup milk
¼ cup nonfat dry milk powder
½ cup cottage cheese
2 tablespoons unsweetened cocoa powder
1 tablespoon toasted wheat germ
1 tablespoon sweetener

Serves 2

Milk, powdered milk, and cottage cheese are all good sources of dietary calcium. Check with your doctor for the latest recommendations on calcium intake during pregnancy. Currently studies suggest that pregnant women take in at least 1,500 mg of calcium per day.

SERVING SIZE: ½ OF RECIPE (325G)			
CALORIES: 220		**CALORIES FROM FAT: 60**	
	%DV*		%DV*
Total Fat 7g	11%	Sugars 21g	
Saturated Fat 4g	20%	Protein 15g	
Cholesterol 20mg	7%	Vitamin A	10%
Sodium 300mg	13%	Vitamin C	0%
Total Carbohydrate 25g	8%	Calcium	30%
Dietary Fiber 2g	8%	Iron	4%
*Percent Daily Values are based on a 2,000 calorie diet			

Cocoa Radical Scavenger

Thick and rich, this chocolaty combination is so delicious you may want to have it every day. The good news is, with all of the health benefits in this one, you can!

1 cup milk
½ cup ice cubes
¼ cup cottage cheese
3 tablespoons unsweetened cocoa powder
2 tablespoons protein powder (such as whey powder)
2 tablespoons peanut butter
1 tablespoon wheat germ

Serves 2

Milk, cottage cheese, and whey contain methionine, which the liver can convert to cysteine, a powerful free-radical scavenger that works with vitamin E to protect cells from degenerative oxidative damage. Wheat germ is also a food source of the amino acid cysteine. Peanuts are an excellent source of vitamin E.

SERVING SIZE: ½ OF RECIPE (242G)			
CALORIES: 250		**CALORIES FROM FAT: 130**	
	%DV*		%DV*
Total Fat 14g	22%	Sugars 9g	
Saturated Fat 4.5g	23%	Protein 18g	
Cholesterol 25mg	8%	Vitamin A	4%
Sodium 240mg	10%	Vitamin C	0%
Total Carbohydrate 16g	5%	Calcium	20%
Dietary Fiber 4g	16%	Iron	6%
*Percent Daily Values are based on a 2,000 calorie diet			

Mineral Booster

Whip up this creamy almond delight when you need an energy boost. It makes taking your minerals every day much less of a chore!

1 cup almond milk
¼ cup pumpkin seeds
¼ cup protein powder
2 tablespoons almond butter
½ teaspoon magnesium powder

Serves 2

During pregnancy, your body needs much more magnesium, calcium, protein, and zinc than usual. Magnesium is a cofactor in more than three hundred enzymatic reactions and is necessary for the transfer, storage, and utilization of energy, and for the production of protein. I use Mama Calm magnesium powder for my pregnant clients. Zinc deficiency is a common cause of fatigue, especially in pregnant women. Pumpkin seeds are one of the richest vegan sources of zinc.

SERVING SIZE: ½ OF RECIPE (175G)			
CALORIES: 320		**CALORIES FROM FAT: 210**	
	%DV*		%DV*
Total Fat 23g	35%	Sugars 5g	
Saturated Fat 3.5g	18%	Protein 20g	
Cholesterol 15mg	5%	Vitamin A	8%
Sodium 170mg	7%	Vitamin C	2%
Total Carbohydrate 12g	4%	Calcium	25%
Dietary Fiber 2g	8%	Iron	30%
*Percent Daily Values are based on a 2,000 calorie diet			

Power Snack

Dates are a delicious source of natural sugar. This fresh and subtle concoction packs a whole lot of energy into one glass.

¼ cup dates
½ cup yogurt
¼ cup ground pumpkin seeds
½ cup milk
2 tablespoons protein powder
Optional: ¼ teaspoon vitamin C powder

Serves 2

Yogurt, pumpkin seeds, milk, and protein power provide some of the extra protein needed during pregnancy. Yogurt also helps to soothe pregnant tummies.

SERVING SIZE: ½ OF RECIPE (179G)			
CALORIES: 320		**CALORIES FROM FAT: 130**	
	%DV*		%DV*
Total Fat 14g	22%	Sugars 26g	
Saturated Fat 3.5g	18%	Protein 20g	
Cholesterol 15mg	5%	Vitamin A	10%
Sodium 95mg	4%	Vitamin C	0%
Total Carbohydrate 33g	11%	Calcium	25%
Dietary Fiber 3g	12%	Iron	25%
*Percent Daily Values are based on a 2,000 calorie diet			

Lemon Spritzer

Many women crave citrus fruits when they are pregnant, and this snappy beverage is the perfect solution.

1 cup sparkling water
½ cup ice cubes
1 tablespoon lemon juice
1 tablespoon xylitol
1 teaspoon electrolyte powder
1 teaspoon flaxseed oil

Serves 1

When your lips are chapped or your skin is dry, it is usually because you are dehydrated. To help you absorb the water you drink, take in extra electrolytes, and be sure you are getting enough essential fatty acids on a regular basis. Here, electrolytes are provided in supplement form and the fatty acids are supplied through flaxseed oil.

SERVING SIZE: 1 (379G)			
CALORIES: 45		**CALORIES FROM FAT: 40**	
	%DV*		%DV*
Total Fat 4.5g	7%	Sugars 0g	
Saturated Fat 0g	0%	Protein 0g	
Cholesterol 0mg	0%	Vitamin A	0%
Sodium 5mg	0%	Vitamin C	10%
Total Carbohydrate 1g	0%	Calcium	15%
Dietary Fiber 0g	0%	Iron	0%
*Percent Daily Values are based on a 2,000 calorie diet			

Soy Iced Coffee

This decaffeinated cold coffee whip is sweet and refreshing.

1 cup decaf coffee
½ cup soymilk
2 cups ice cubes
1 teaspoon vanilla extract
1 teaspoon sweetener
¼ teaspoon magnesium powder

Serves 1

Instant coffees can be added as crystals directly to your drink. Pregnant women should avoid caffeine whenever possible. The use of soymilk provides additional protein.

SERVING SIZE: 1 (845G)			
CALORIES: 100		**CALORIES FROM FAT: 20**	
	%DV*		%DV*
Total Fat 2.5g	4%	Sugars 6g	
Saturated Fat 0g	0%	Protein 6g	
Cholesterol 0mg	0%	Vitamin A	15%
Sodium 90mg	4%	Vitamin C	0%
Total Carbohydrate 12g	4%	Calcium	6%
Dietary Fiber 2g	8%	Iron	8%
*Percent Daily Values are based on a 2,000 calorie diet			

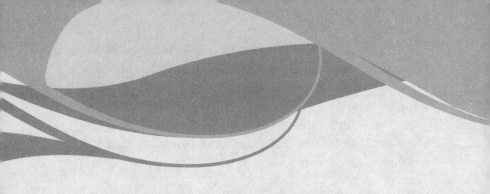

...Children and Infants...

When it comes to delivering vitamins and minerals, smoothies are an easy sell with the younger set. Smoothies for kids can take many forms. They can be rich and creamy, reminiscent of milkshakes, sweet and flavorful with a hint of culinary spices, or they can be light and refreshing like lemonade or your child's favorite soda.

Children are known for being some of the pickiest people on earth. This may be because they have not yet become familiar enough with the plethora of foods available to trust all of them. They tend to stick to the foods they know, which can greatly restrict their nutrient intake. For example, it is not uncommon for children to go through long phases of wanting only pasta, cold cereal, dairy products, or fruit. During these phases they may be missing out on several important nutritional components essential for their growth and development.

Some of the nutrient categories that can become challenging for children are the protein needed for cellular development, minerals needed for bones, B vitamins that are critical for hormone and enzyme production, and omega-3 fatty acids that are necessary for brain and neurological development.

Another aspect of children's nutrition to keep in mind is that overconsumption of processed and fast foods, which are full of excess sodium, food coloring, refined carbohydrates, sugar, and saturated fats, can be devastating to your child's health. The smoothies in this chapter, however, meet many of the nutritional needs of today's children and can be equally fast, and more fun to prepare, than fast food or packaged goods.

General Nutrition Guidelines

Just as many of us have special dietary preferences or needs, such as food allergies that restrict certain foods from our diet, some children's diets demand an equal level of sophistication. Many parents may have already identified that sugar, for example, causes their children to feel cranky and out of control, or that synthetic food dyes affect their ability to concentrate. Therefore, it is up to the shopper in the house to encourage each child's understanding of his or her own health needs and support them in creating smoothies that satisfy their culinary peculiarities and nutritional needs.

Nutritionally speaking, the motto in your house should be "The more colorful, the better." In the world of plant foods, such as fruits and vegetables, the color you see is actually derived from nutrients such as vitamins and minerals. So by choosing colorful whole foods for your children's drinks, you can be sure that you are providing nutrient-dense snacks and meals.

The following nutrients are especially important for children, and many are available in multiple foods to satisfy even the really picky eaters who may be missing out on one or more nutrients needed for proper growth.

Cholesterol

Cholesterol is found in all animal products in varying degrees. Although this fatty substance can become a problem if too much adheres to the blood vessels, it is a necessary nutrient for many bodily functions, including growth hormone production. Food sources include milk, yogurt, cottage cheese, and ice cream.

Water

To determine a child's water need, divide his or her weight in half. This gives you a guideline for the minimum number of ounces of water the child needs in order to stay hydrated. For example, a child who weighs 60 pounds needs to drink at least 30 ounces (3½ glasses) of fresh water each day. Adding filtered water, sparkling water, or ice to smoothies increases water content. If your child does not drink enough water, this is a good strategy for increasing overall intake.

Electrolytes

Minerals such as calcium, magnesium, sodium, and potassium are necessary for the conduction of electrical currents throughout the body. They can be added to smoothies in liquid or powdered form.

Protein

Children often have a hard time getting the protein they need, as eating habits often tend toward carbohydrate-based foods such as pasta and cereal. Food sources include nuts, seeds, nut butter, and dairy foods such as yogurt, milk, nonfat dry milk, cottage cheese, and soy foods such as tofu and soymilk. Delicious protein powders are also available to add to smoothies and are virtually undetectable. The following is a general guideline.

AGE	DAILY CALORIES	PROTEIN (grams)
1–3	1,300 (900–1,800)	23
4–6	1,700 (1,300–2,300)	30
7–10	2,400 (1,650–3,000)	34

Dairy

Always buy organic yogurt, milk, cheese, and ice cream for children. Unless they are organic, dairy products can contain any number of antibiotics, hormones, pesticides, or herbicides.

- **Milk** Buy whole milk for children unless they are overweight, in which case 2 percent milk is a good choice. Organic chocolate milk is often available in grocery stores. Nonfat dry milk powder adds more than 1 gram of protein per tablespoon and adds a creamy richness to smoothies that kids love.
- **Yogurt** Look for yogurt that does not contain food coloring, corn syrup, synthetic sweeteners, or chemical preservatives. There are plenty of health-conscious yogurt makers, such as Stonyfield Farm, who produce organic yogurt with natural colors and sweeteners and use only fresh fruit.
- **Whey powder** Whey powder is high in protein and also includes nutrients that help remove heavy metals and many toxins from the body.
- **Cottage cheese** Cottage cheese hides nicely in smoothies because it blends so well and becomes creamy almost instantly.

Fruit

Use organic fruits whenever possible. Feel free to experiment with a variety of textures to find the ones that appeal to your child, such as purees like applesauce, juices, fresh whole or sliced fruit, frozen fruit (especially bananas and seasonal fruit such as berries and mangoes), and canned or jarred fruit.

Probiotics

These healthy bacteria colonize in the gut, giving the entire 20-foot-long digestive tract a protective layer. Probiotics are supplements that help build healthy levels of microflora in the digestive tract, which protect us from bad bacteria, viruses, organisms that cause food poisoning, and unhealthy yeasts. Many yogurt products are infused with probiotics, and microflora (probiotics) can be purchased in powdered form.

Sweeteners

Use natural sweeteners such as molasses, jam, xylitol, agave syrup, brown rice syrup, barley malt syrup, stevia, honey, and turbinado (unrefined cane sugar). Avoid synthetic sweeteners like aspartame, saccharin, and sucralose, which have been linked to cancer development in animal subjects.

Now it's time for some fun. After you try these delicious concoctions, use them as inspiration to make up your own recipes. Ask your kids what flavors they love, like strawberry milkshake, cheesecake, or Key lime pie, and then use those flavors to create the basis of their drinks. Add in the nutrients they need—a scoop of protein powder, ¼ teaspoon of electrolyte powder, or 1 tablespoon of flaxseed oil would do it. If they drink nutritionally designed smoothies such as these daily, smoothies can become a vehicle for nutrients like calcium to help bones and nails to grow strong, oils to keep hair shiny, minerals that assist in sustaining energy, and protein that supports muscle development. It's also a good way to bond with your children and introduce them to tasty new treats!

Lemon Sparkle

Reminiscent of carbonated lemonade, Lemon Sparkle has a tart, fizzy flavor that makes it a perfect lunchtime pick-me-up.

2 cups sparkling water
¼ teaspoon electrolyte powder
1–2 teaspoons sweetener
1 tablespoon lemon juice

Serves 2

If you or your kids have a hard time getting enough water each day, this refreshing drink might be just the ticket. It's full of electrolytes that help your body absorb water. Our brains work much better and we have more energy when we are well hydrated.

SERVING SIZE: ½ OF RECIPE (248G)			
CALORIES: 15		**CALORIES FROM FAT: 0**	
	%DV*		%DV*
Total Fat 0g	0%	Sugars 3g	
Saturated Fat 0g	0%	Protein 0g	
Cholesterol 0mg	0%	Vitamin A	0%
Sodium 10mg	0%	Vitamin C	6%
Total Carbohydrate 3g	1%	Calcium	4%
Dietary Fiber 0g	0%	Iron	0%
*Percent Daily Values are based on a 2,000 calorie diet			

Peanut Butter Cup

What kid doesn't love peanut butter candy? This rich dessert will make your children feel truly luxuriant.

1 cup milk
1 cup vanilla yogurt
2 tablespoons unsweetened cocoa powder
¼ cup ice cubes
2 tablespoons nut butter (macadamia, creamy peanut butter, etc.)
2 tablespoons nonfat dried milk powder
1 teaspoon vanilla extract

Serves 2

This high-protein treat packs a load of antioxidants from the cocoa powder and healthful probiotics from the yogurt, which is good for digestion.

SERVING SIZE: ½ OF RECIPE (292G)			
CALORIES: 270		**CALORIES FROM FAT: 130**	
	%DV*		%DV*
Total Fat 14g	22%	Sugars 17g	
Saturated Fat 5g	25%	Protein 15g	
Cholesterol 20mg	7%	Vitamin A	8%
Sodium 230mg	10%	Vitamin C	2%
Total Carbohydrate 22g	7%	Calcium	40%
Dietary Fiber 2g	8%	Iron	4%
*Percent Daily Values are based on a 2,000 calorie diet			

Peppermint Cream

Nothing says childhood like peppermint candy.

1 cup milk
1 cup ice cubes
½ cup ice cream
½ cup plain yogurt
1 drop peppermint oil

Serves 2

Peppermint stimulates bile flow and aids in digestion. Children are often under stress from their busy schedules, which results in stomachaches from maldigestion of food. A daily smoothie for digestion may help them absorb their nutrients and give them more energy throughout the day.

SERVING SIZE: ½ OF RECIPE (330G)			
CALORIES: 170		**CALORIES FROM FAT: 70**	
	%DV*		%DV*
Total Fat 8g	12%	Sugars 17g	
Saturated Fat 4.5g	23%	Protein 9g	
Cholesterol 30mg	10%	Vitamin A	10%
Sodium 135mg	6%	Vitamin C	0%
Total Carbohydrate 18g	6%	Calcium	30%
Dietary Fiber 0g	0%	Iron	0%
*Percent Daily Values are based on a 2,000 calorie diet			

Nap Time

Sweet and creamy with a hint of maple, this smoothie works well as part of a ritual to prepare for sleeping.

1 cup milk
1 frozen peeled banana
½ cup frozen pitted cherries
¼ cup nonfat dry milk powder
1 tablespoon maple syrup
1 teaspoon grated nutmeg

Serves 2

Milk contains tryptophan, which is the amino acid known for inducing sleep. This is the perfect pre-nap or pre-bedtime drink.

SERVING SIZE: ½ OF RECIPE (239G)			
CALORIES: 210		**CALORIES FROM FAT: 45**	
	%DV*		%DV*
Total Fat 4.5g	7%	Sugars 27g	
Saturated Fat 2.5g	13%	Protein 8g	
Cholesterol 15mg	5%	Vitamin A	15%
Sodium 100mg	4%	Vitamin C	10%
Total Carbohydrate 35g	12%	Calcium	25%
Dietary Fiber 2g	8%	Iron	4%
*Percent Daily Values are based on a 2,000 calorie diet			

Fruit Power for the Vegetabley Impaired

With its deep purple color and juicy flavor, this smoothie is fun to drink!

1 cup pomegranate juice
1 cup frozen blueberries
1 banana, fresh or frozen, peeled
Optional: frozen apple, or grape juice concentrate, or honey as sweetener

Serves 2

Those who aren't getting enough fresh vegetables need not worry, as many of the same nutrients found in vegetables are also found in some fruits. This combination is chock full of antioxidants, vitamins, and minerals.

SERVING SIZE: ½ OF RECIPE (263G)			
CALORIES: 160		**CALORIES FROM FAT: 5**	
	%DV*		%DV*
Total Fat 0.5g	1%	Sugars 31g	
Saturated Fat 0g	0%	Protein 1g	
Cholesterol 0mg	0%	Vitamin A	2%
Sodium 15mg	1%	Vitamin C	10%
Total Carbohydrate 40g	13%	Calcium	2%
Dietary Fiber 4g	16%	Iron	2%
*Percent Daily Values are based on a 2,000 calorie diet			

Bubbly Fruit Cooler

Pineapple adds a special zing to any drink. Just be sure to blend it until smooth or your straw will be useless. You can also use tropical juice, if preferred.

1½ cups frozen tropical fruit
1½ cups ginger ale (see Note)
½ cup pineapple or orange sherbet

Serves 2

Use fresh or canned tropical fruit and add the juice from the can to the smoothie.

Tropical fruits are excellent sources of vitamin C and carotenoids such as beta-carotene, which protects the skin from the sun's ultraviolet light.

NOTE: Add sparkling water instead of ginger ale to make this less sweet.

SERVING SIZE: ½ OF RECIPE (360G)			
CALORIES: 210		**CALORIES FROM FAT: 5**	
	%DV*		%DV*
Total Fat 0.5g	1%	Sugars 46g	
Saturated Fat 0g	0%	Protein 1g	
Cholesterol 0mg	0%	Vitamin A	20%
Sodium 30mg	1%	Vitamin C	60%
Total Carbohydrate 51g	17%	Calcium	2%
Dietary Fiber 4g	16%	Iron	2%
*Percent Daily Values are based on a 2,000 calorie diet			

Coconut Cream Frosty

If you are crazy for coconut, you will love this thick, tropical delight. Add Perrier for a less sweet, lighter version.

1 cup milk
½ cup coconut juice or coconut water
½ cup ice cubes
3 tablespoons nonfat dry milk powder or cottage cheese
Optional: ¼ cup grated coconut

Serves 2

Coconut juice is an excellent source of electrolytes. Milk and cottage cheese also provide protein, and additional ice helps hydrate the body.

SERVING SIZE: ½ OF RECIPE (248G)			
CALORIES: 110		**CALORIES FROM FAT: 35**	
	%DV*		%DV*
Total Fat 4g	6%	Sugars 10g	
Saturated Fat 2.5g	13%	Protein 7g	
Cholesterol 15mg	5%	Vitamin A	6%
Sodium 150mg	6%	Vitamin C	2%
Total Carbohydrate 11g	4%	Calcium	25%
Dietary Fiber 1g	4%	Iron	2%
*Percent Daily Values are based on a 2,000 calorie diet			

Watermelon Spritzer

This is the simplest smoothie ever. Just add watermelon and you've got a summery treat for even the pickiest palate.

1 cup seedless watermelon
Optional: 1 cup sparkling water
         ¼ teaspoon electrolyte powder

Serves 1

Watermelon happens to be a rich source of carotenoids that protect the skin from cancer. So drink up before a day at the pool, or out in the playfield to protect skin and eyes.

SERVING SIZE: 1 (152G)			
CALORIES: 45		**CALORIES FROM FAT: 0**	
	%DV*		%DV*
Total Fat 0g	0%	Sugars 9g	
Saturated Fat 0g	0%	Protein 1g	
Cholesterol 0mg	0%	Vitamin A	15%
Sodium 0mg	0%	Vitamin C	20%
Total Carbohydrate 11g	4%	Calcium	2%
Dietary Fiber 1g	4%	Iron	2%
*Percent Daily Values are based on a 2,000 calorie diet			

Grump Be Gone

Put a smile on your children's faces with a crisp, shimmery concoction designed to pick up their energy levels.

1 cup apple juice
¼ cup frozen apple juice concentrate
⅓ cup nonfat dry milk powder
1 cup frozen peaches

Serves 2

This is a magic formula for bringing up low blood sugar levels. The apple juice offers a quick infusion of healthy fruit sugar while the milk powder serves up 4 grams of protein to banish the low blood sugar blues.

SERVING SIZE: ½ OF RECIPE (234G)			
CALORIES: 170		**CALORIES FROM FAT: 0**	
	%DV*		%DV*
Total Fat 0g	0%	Sugars 37g	
Saturated Fat 0g	0%	Protein 5g	
Cholesterol 0mg	0%	Vitamin A	8%
Sodium 70mg	3%	Vitamin C	120%
Total Carbohydrate 39g	13%	Calcium	15%
Dietary Fiber 1g	4%	Iron	4%
*Percent Daily Values are based on a 2,000 calorie diet			

Smile Maker

Strawberries and apple juice whipped together with a frozen banana give this frosty a thick texture. This is perfect for picky eaters who are wary of new foods.

1 cup frozen strawberries
½ cup apple juice
1 frozen peeled banana

Serves 1

Strawberries are an excellent fruit choice for children who are sensitive to sugar, as they contain a special fiber that slows the release of the fruit sugars into the body.

SERVING SIZE: 1 (391G)			
CALORIES: 210		**CALORIES FROM FAT: 5**	
	%DV*		%DV*
Total Fat 0.5g	1%	Sugars 35g	
Saturated Fat 0g	0%	Protein 2g	
Cholesterol 0mg	0%	Vitamin A	2%
Sodium 0mg	0%	Vitamin C	120%
Total Carbohydrate 55g	18%	Calcium	2%
Dietary Fiber 6g	24%	Iron	8%
*Percent Daily Values are based on a 2,000 calorie diet			

The Tired Treatment

This refreshing bubbly punch sits lightly on the stomach and is perfect before athletic endeavors or an afternoon playing outside.

1 cup sparkling water
1 cup ice cubes
½ cup ginger ale
½ cup frozen lemonade concentrate
¼ teaspoon electrolyte powder

Serves 2

The water content in this smoothie is very high, and the ginger ale has just enough sugar to help carry the minerals from the electrolyte powder into the bloodstream to rehydrate and replenish blood sugar levels.

SERVING SIZE: ½ OF RECIPE (371G)			
CALORIES: 150		**CALORIES FROM FAT: 0**	
	%DV*		%DV*
Total Fat 0g	0%	Sugars 35g	
Saturated Fat 0g	0%	Protein 0g	
Cholesterol 0mg	0%	Vitamin A	0%
Sodium 15mg	1%	Vitamin C	20%
Total Carbohydrate 40g	3%	Calcium	4%
Dietary Fiber 0g	0%	Iron	4%
*Percent Daily Values are based on a 2,000 calorie diet			

Calming Cooler

Smooth and subtle, bananas and almonds are guaranteed to help little ones relax and calm down.

1 cup almond milk
1 frozen peeled banana
2 tablespoons almond butter
¼ teaspoon magnesium

Serves 1

Magnesium helps relax the body. Nuts such as almonds contain magnesium and milk contains tryptophan, the amino acid known for relaxing the mind and body.

SERVING SIZE: 1 (391G)			
CALORIES: 370		**CALORIES FROM FAT: 200**	
	%DV*		%DV*
Total Fat 22g	34%	Sugars 23g	
Saturated Fat 2g	10%	Protein 7g	
Cholesterol 0mg	0%	Vitamin A	15%
Sodium 290mg	12%	Vitamin C	15%
Total Carbohydrate 42g	14%	Calcium	30%
Dietary Fiber 5g	20%	Iron	10%
*Percent Daily Values are based on a 2,000 calorie diet			

...Baby Smoothies...

Ask your pediatrician when you can introduce solid food into your child's diet. Newborn babies have permeable digestive tracts, which function best with mother's milk. Around six months, when teeth begin to appear, their digestive tract is fully formed and ready for the introduction of pureed whole foods, such as cooked vegetables and fruits. Slowly introduce new produce, so that if your child has a reaction to a particular food it will be easier to identify what caused the reaction. Also, be sure all foods are organic.

Ichiban

Bananas are naturally sweet and when frozen before blending, they give smoothies a milkshake texture.

½ cup Rice & Soy Beverage
½ frozen peeled banana
½ teaspoon vanilla extract
2 tablespoons unsweetened organic cocoa powder

Serves 1

Use rice protein powder for babies who are sensitive or allergic to dairy. I used Eden Blend Rice & Soy Beverage because it's so creamy and makes perfect smoothies. The Dagoba unsweetened cocoa is high in antioxidants.

SERVING SIZE: 1 (192G)			
CALORIES: 150		**CALORIES FROM FAT: 25**	
	%DV*		%DV*
Total Fat 2.5g	4%	Sugars 11g	
Saturated Fat 0g	0%	Protein 6g	
Cholesterol 0mg	0%	Vitamin A	0%
Sodium 45mg	2%	Vitamin C	8%
Total Carbohydrate 29g	10%	Calcium	2%
Dietary Fiber 4g	16%	Iron	8%
*Percent Daily Values are based on a 2,000 calorie diet			

Baby's Favorite

In babies polled, this combination was the five-star favorite.

½ cup milk
½ avocado, peeled and pitted
½ banana, peeled
2 tablespoons nonfat dry milk powder

Serves 1

Babies love this combination and you can feel good about feeding it to them every day. Milk and milk powder provide protein, avocados are an excellent source of essential fatty acids, and the banana contains electrolytes.

SERVING SIZE: 1 (290G)			
CALORIES: 320		**CALORIES FROM FAT: 170**	
	%DV*		%DV*
Total Fat 19g	29%	Sugars 18g	
Saturated Fat 4.5g	23%	Protein 10g	
Cholesterol 15mg	5%	Vitamin A	10%
Sodium 105mg	4%	Vitamin C	25%
Total Carbohydrate 32g	11%	Calcium	25%
Dietary Fiber 8g	32%	Iron	4%
*Percent Daily Values are based on a 2,000 calorie diet			

Apple Cream

This one is a natural for babies as it marries their natural proclivity for dairy with the interesting flavor of apples.

½ cup ice cubes
½ cup apple juice concentrate
2 tablespoons cottage cheese
1 teaspoon flaxseed oil

Serves 1

Apple juice provides fruit sugar, cottage cheese is an amazingly dense source of protein, and flaxseed oil provides some of the essential fatty acids a baby needs for nerve and brain development.

SERVING SIZE: 1 (265G)			
CALORIES: 250		**CALORIES FROM FAT: 50**	
	%DV*		%DV*
Total Fat 6g	9%	Sugars 45g	
Saturated Fat 1g	5%	Protein 4g	
Cholesterol 5mg	2%	Vitamin A	2%
Sodium 135mg	6%	Vitamin C	4%
Total Carbohydrate 47g	16%	Calcium	6%
Dietary Fiber 0g	0%	Iron	6%
*Percent Daily Values are based on a 2,000 calorie diet			

Brain Food

Of course, most babies go bananas for ... well ... bananas. So if you're going to start making smoothies for your child, Brain Food might be a good place to start.

½ cup milk
½ frozen peeled banana
2 tablespoons cottage cheese
1 teaspoon flavored fish oil

Serves 1

Some nutritional-supplement companies make yummy kid's cod liver oil products, which are perfect for smoothies. Babies' brains and nervous systems need the fatty acids from plants and from fish to develop properly. Cottage cheese is a concentrated source of protein that blends so well in smoothies that it gives drinks a cream-like texture. Bananas provide electrolytes to support hydration.

SERVING SIZE: 1 (214G)			
CALORIES: 190		**CALORIES FROM FAT: 90**	
	%DV*		%DV*
Total Fat 10g	15%	Sugars 14g	
Saturated Fat 4g	20%	Protein 8g	
Cholesterol 40mg	13%	Vitamin A	100%
Sodium 150mg	6%	Vitamin C	8%
Total Carbohydrate 20g	7%	Calcium	15%
Dietary Fiber 2g	8%	Iron	2%
*Percent Daily Values are based on a 2,000 calorie diet			

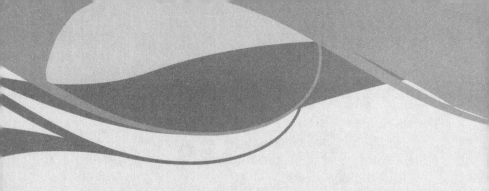

...Home Barista Guide...

There is a whole kitchen coffee culture brewing that is bringing people home from the coffee shops. These home brewers are capitalizing on the opportunity to luxuriate in their own homes, with their friends, their music, and their favorite ingredients to create luscious cold coffee drinks that are actually healthy.

Even better, these coffee smoothies will not let you crash, as you do from a regular cup of joe, as they contain nutrients to balance the adrenal rush you get from the caffeine.

Barista Ingredient Primer

Coffee

Choose a coffee that is organic, if possible, because organic coffees tend to have higher antioxidant levels. You can bring home whole beans and grind them in a coffee grinder or food processor, or have them ground and store the ground coffee in an airtight bag to keep it fresh.

To brew your coffee, use either a French press, a paper-filter system (manual or automatic), or an espresso steamer. You can also cold-brew, which makes sweet coffee with fewer bitter compounds. This is the Toddy method and uses 1 pound of fresh-ground coffee, 2 quarts fresh water, and a simple filtration system. The mixture sits for 12 to 24 hours. The coffee is delicious. Both brewed and cold-drip coffee can be stored in the refrigerator for up to a week.

Instant coffee is simply brewed coffee that has been freeze-dried. There are organic dried products available now that taste so much better than the products our grandparents used to drink.

Coffee Substitutes

Products such as Postum, Bambu, Pero, Roastaroma, Teeccino, and Cafix are all known as coffee substitutes. They are made from ingredients such as roasted chicory, wheat, malted barley, rye, roasted barley, and roasted carob, with the addition of spices such as cinnamon, allspice, and star anise.

Extracts and Oils

Extracts add a whole lot of flavor without the sugar contained in most syrups. Use real, not synthetic, extracts such as vanilla, hazelnut, almond, orange, mint, peppermint, coconut, or banana.

Essential oils add big flavor and aromatic depth to smoothies without adding calories or excessive fats—just a drop or two per glass is enough. Many oils are available at mainstream grocery stores, and include common cinnamon oil, anise, clove, ginger, grapefruit, lavender, lemon, lime, orange, peppermint, rose, spearmint, tangerine, and wintergreen.

Malt

When grain seeds start to grow into plants, it is called sprouting. At this point in the plant's growth, much of the grain's starch has converted to sugar. When sprouts are roasted to caramelize the sugar, malt is produced. Most of us are familiar with the flavor of malt from malted milkshakes. Malt extract powder is made from malted barley and is rich in nutritional value, containing minerals such as magnesium and potassium, essential amino acids, folic acid, and vitamins, particularly vitamin B.

Milk

Whether buying 1 percent, 2 percent, whole, half-and-half, cream, or dried milk powder, always try to buy organic dairy products to avoid hormones such as BGH (bovine growth hormone), chemical residues, and genetically modified organisms.

Spices

Ground spices such as nutmeg, cinnamon, cloves, cardamom, anise, allspice, Chinese five-spice (cinnamon, fennel, star anise, cloves, and Sichuan pepper), coriander, ginger, fennel, and cocoa powder are all delicious in coffee-based smoothies. Chai spice mixes can be used individually and include cloves, cinnamon, nutmeg, ginger, cardamom, and pepper.

Sweeteners

To sweeten drinks, use small quantities of healthful whole ingredients such as agave syrup, maple syrup, barley malt, and honey (liquid or dried) or the alcohol sweeteners such as xylitol, maltitol, malitol, sorbitol, and the herbal sweeteners such as stevia, or chicory sweeteners such as Just Like Sugar.

Tea

There are many types of exotic and healthful teas available today. Experiment until you find the teas that you like best, brew them, and store the prepared tea for up to four days in the refrigerator in a glass pitcher. You will then have tea on hand to add to tea-based smoothies at a whim. Try white, green, black, red (Roibos), oolong, yerba mate, chamomile, chai, peppermint, passion fruit, anise, licorice, genmaicha, mugicha, ginger, lemongrass, toasted rice tea, and rose hip tea.

Frapoothie

Trust me—a Frapoothie is as fun to drink as it is to say out loud. The ice turns this into a thick coffee-flavored slushee.

1 cup decaf coffee
1 cup ice cubes
1 cup milk
2 tablespoons nonfat dry milk powder
1 teaspoon Just Like Sugar or other natural
   sweetener

Serves 2

Researchers found that women who drank more than six cups a day of any type of coffee were 22 percent less likely to develop type 2 diabetes—the kind that occurs in adult life—compared to those who avoided coffee. But diabetes risk dropped even more—by 33 percent—for those who drank more than six cups a day of decaf.

SERVING SIZE: ½ OF RECIPE (363G)			
CALORIES: 90		**CALORIES FROM FAT: 35**	
	%DV*		%DV*
Total Fat 4g	6%	Sugars 8g	
Saturated Fat 2.5g	13%	Protein 6g	
Cholesterol 15mg	5%	Vitamin A	4%
Sodium 80mg	3%	Vitamin C	0%
Total Carbohydrate 8g	3%	Calcium	20%
Dietary Fiber 0g	0%	Iron	0%
*Percent Daily Values are based on a 2,000 calorie diet			

Creamy Café au Lait

This drink is dreamy in flavor and texture.

1 cup coffee
1 cup milk
½ cup ice cubes
⅓ cup nonfat dry milk powder
½ teaspoon vanilla extract
Optional: 1 teaspoon sweetener
       1 tablespoon unsweetened cocoa powder

Serves 1

As a daily coffee drink, this smoothie is much better for you than plain coffee, in that the dry milk powder adds 8 grams of protein, which helps stabilize blood sugar for hours.

SERVING SIZE: 1 (624G)			
CALORIES: 240		**CALORIES FROM FAT: 70**	
	%DV*		%DV*
Total Fat 8g	12%	Sugars 23g	
Saturated Fat 4.5g	23%	Protein 16g	
Cholesterol 25mg	8%	Vitamin A	15%
Sodium 230mg	10%	Vitamin C	2%
Total Carbohydrate 23g	8%	Calcium	60%
Dietary Fiber 0g	0%	Iron	0%
*Percent Daily Values are based on a 2,000 calorie diet			

Honey Iced Macchiato

Macchiato, is pronounced mah-kee-YAH-toe.

1 cup instant coffee crystals
1 cup milk
1 cup ice cubes
1 tablespoon honey
1 teaspoon vanilla extract

Serves 1

Add protein powder to this morning drink to help stabilize blood sugar and provide fuel for your body throughout the day.

SERVING SIZE: 1 (550G)			
CALORIES: 330		**CALORIES FROM FAT: 70**	
	%DV*		%DV*
Total Fat 8g	12%	Sugars 28g	
Saturated Fat 4.5g	23%	Protein 13g	
Cholesterol 25mg	8%	Vitamin A	4%
Sodium 125mg	5%	Vitamin C	0%
Total Carbohydrate 46g	15%	Calcium	35%
Dietary Fiber 0g	0%	Iron	10%
*Percent Daily Values are based on a 2,000 calorie diet			

Iced Mocha Valencia

Few people know that the vast cultivation of the Valencia orange in California led to the naming of Orange County. Today, the word *Valencia* is interchangable with orange, such was the popularity of this strain. You'll be surprised at how much even a little orange flavoring can perk up your morning coffee.

1 cup brewed or drip coffee
1 cup milk
½ cup ice cubes
2 tablespoons unsweetened organic cocoa powder
5 drops orange extract
Optional: Valencia (orange) syrup

Serves 1

Other extracts and oils can be used in place of the orange extract—peppermint and vanilla are two of my favorite substitutes.

SERVING SIZE: 1 (610G)			
CALORIES: 180		**CALORIES FROM FAT: 80**	
	%DV*		%DV*
Total Fat 9g	14%	Sugars 11g	
Saturated Fat 4.5g	23%	Protein 10g	
Cholesterol 25mg	8%	Vitamin A	4%
Sodium 105mg	4%	Vitamin C	0%
Total Carbohydrate 17g	6%	Calcium	30%
Dietary Fiber 2g	8%	Iron	4%
*Percent Daily Values are based on a 2,000 calorie diet			

Vanilla Crème Freeze

By making coffee drinks at home, you can subtly alter the flavors and sweetener to create your perfect blend. That said, any mixture of the following ingredients is bound to please anyone!

1 cup strong coffee
½ cup milk
½ cup ice cubes
¼ cup nonfat dry milk powder
1 teaspoon vanilla extract
1 teaspoon sweetener
Optional: ½ teaspoon mint or orange extract

Serves 1

This traditionally cold, blended drink is a healthier version of a coffee milkshake. The nonfat dry milk adds more than 6 grams of protein and the vanilla extract adds flavor without much sugar.

SERVING SIZE: 1 (506G)			
CALORIES: 170		**CALORIES FROM FAT: 35**	
	%DV*		%DV*
Total Fat 4g	6%	Sugars 20g	
Saturated Fat 2.5g	13%	Protein 10g	
Cholesterol 15mg	5%	Vitamin A	10%
Sodium 150mg	6%	Vitamin C	2%
Total Carbohydrate 21g	7%	Calcium	35%
Dietary Fiber 0g	0%	Iron	0%
*Percent Daily Values are based on a 2,000 calorie diet			

Malted Café au Lait

Adding malt to coffee drinks brings to mind the malted milk drinks of childhood. This is a good way to start each day with a smile on your face.

1 cup coffee
1 cup milk
½ cup ice cubes
¼ cup nonfat dry milk powder
1 tablespoon malted milk powder

Serves 1

Nonfat dried milk powder gives you a little boost of extra protein, which will stabilize your blood sugar and give you energy throughout the day.

SERVING SIZE: 1 (638G)				
CALORIES: 300		**CALORIES FROM FAT: 90**		
	%DV*			%DV*
Total Fat 10g	15%	Sugars 30g		
Saturated Fat 6g	30%	Protein 17g		
Cholesterol 30mg	10%	Vitamin A		15%
Sodium 290mg	12%	Vitamin C		2%
Total Carbohydrate 35g	12%	Calcium		60%
Dietary Fiber 0g	0%	Iron		2%
*Percent Daily Values are based on a 2,000 calorie diet				

Green Cream Tea

If you prefer a subtle green tea flavor, steep the tea leaves for just under two minutes. Studies have shown that this is all the time you need to fully infuse the hot water with the leaves' medicinal properties.

1 cup green tea
1 cup milk
½ cup ice cubes
¼ cup nonfat dry milk powder
1 tablespoon sweetener
Optional: 2 tablespoons dried, instant green tea flakes

Serves 1

The catechin polyphenols in green tea raise thermogenesis (the rate at which calories are burned), thus increasing the availability of energy and speeding up your metabolism.

SERVING SIZE: 1 (637G)			
CALORIES: 280		**CALORIES FROM FAT: 70**	
	%DV*		%DV*
Total Fat 8g	12%	Sugars 36g	
Saturated Fat 4.5g	23%	Protein 14g	
Cholesterol 25mg	8%	Vitamin A	15%
Sodium 200mg	8%	Vitamin C	2%
Total Carbohydrate 37g	12%	Calcium	50%
Dietary Fiber 0g	0%	Iron	0%
*Percent Daily Values are based on a 2,000 calorie diet			

Chai Crème Frappé

In Hindi, *chai* is simply the word for "tea." In English, however, the term generally refers to a specific tea, Masala Chai, which is a spicy combination of cardamom, cinnamon, ginger, star anise, peppercorn, and cloves.

1 cup Chai tea
1 cup milk
½ cup ice cubes
¼ cup nonfat dry milk powder
1 tablespoon honey

Serves 2

Spices such as cardamom, ginger, and cinnamon are used in Ayurvedic medicine to increase energy and balance many of the body's systems. Nonfat dry milk will definitely increase energy, as it provides needed protein early in the day.

SERVING SIZE: ½ OF RECIPE (319G)			
CALORIES: 140		**CALORIES FROM FAT: 35**	
	%DV*		%DV*
Total Fat 4g	6%	Sugars 18g	
Saturated Fat 2.5g	13%	Protein 7g	
Cholesterol 15mg	5%	Vitamin A	6%
Sodium 100mg	4%	Vitamin C	0%
Total Carbohydrate 19g	6%	Calcium	25%
Dietary Fiber 0g	0%	Iron	0%
*Percent Daily Values are based on a 2,000 calorie diet			

Cold Brevé

Cold espresso drinks, also known as igloo espresso, originated in Italy. The term *brevé* simply refers to an espresso
drink made with half-and-half.

2 teaspoons instant decaf coffee crystals
¼ cup boiling water
½ cup half-and-half
½ cup ice cubes
2 tablespoons nonfat dry milk powder

Serves 1

Mix the instant coffee crystals in hot water to dissolve. Pour
the coffee into the blender and add the remaining ingredients. Although half-and-half has more calories than skim
milk, it contains the same nutrients and creates a much
creamier drink.

SERVING SIZE: 1 (310G)			
CALORIES: 190		**CALORIES FROM FAT: 120**	
	%DV*		%DV*
Total Fat 14g	22%	Sugars 5g	
Saturated Fat 9g	45%	Protein 7g	
Cholesterol 45mg	15%	Vitamin A	10%
Sodium 105mg	4%	Vitamin C	2%
Total Carbohydrate 11g	4%	Calcium	25%
Dietary Fiber 0g	0%	Iron	2%
*Percent Daily Values are based on a 2,000 calorie diet			

healthful smoothies ingredients

Açaí

Pronounced ah-SIGH-yee, açaí is a delicious Amazonian berry that comes from a palm tree, like dates. Its nutritional offerings include the omega-6 and omega-9 fatty acids and antioxidants such as vitamin E. Açaí is available in most Western grocery stores as juice or frozen fruit pulp. Some say that the deep purple fruit pulp is reminiscent of a blueberry sorbet or ice cream with a hint of chocolate. Be aware that açaí contains some caffeine and some açaí products contain guarana, which is a stimulant.

Acidophilus

Probiotics such as *Lactobacillus acidophilus* and *Bifidobacterium bifidum*, also known as beneficial microflora or healthy gut bacteria, are essential components of a healthy digestive tract. There are four hundred known organisms that are part of a healthy microflora environment in the intestines. They are capable of protecting our bodies by outcompeting such harmful organisms as *Candida albicans* and *Salmonella* bacteria. Although they can become depleted from the use of antibiotics and alcohol, or the influence of stress-related hormones, you can replace them by eating yogurt, miso, or cultured milk. You can also take live-culture supplements such as acidophilus and bifidus. Probiotic powder is relatively tasteless and blends well in smoothies. Buy the product in its powdered form or open up a capsule and pour the contents into the blender and discard the gel capsule.

Almonds

Sliced or chopped almonds can be incorporated into smoothies to add fiber and protein as well as magnesium, riboflavin, and vitamin E. Research has revealed nine phenolic compounds in almonds, of which eight exhibit strong antioxidant activity.

Amasake

Amasake is a traditional Japanese product made from fermented sweet brown rice. It is a creamy beverage that can be used in smoothies and other drinks as a sweetener.

Apples

Apples are a good source of the soluble fiber pectin, which is helpful in cholesterol regulation and blood sugar control. In the intestine, apple pectin is a bulk-forming agent similar to psyllium. Pectin may modify intestinal bacterial enzyme activity in favor of a reduction of toxic breakdown products in the gut.

Apples are also a good source of polyphenols, which are known for their anti-microbial action and infection-prevention abilities; glutathione, a potent antioxidant that helps prevent heart disease and cancer; and malic acid, a fruit acid that is a powerful binder of heavy metals such as cadmium and lead.

Be sure to choose organic apples, as apples are often a heavily sprayed crop. Always core your apples before blending, and either skin them or finely blend them if you leave the skins on.

Apple Juice

Look for unsweetened apple juice to avoid added sugars. Apple works well in smoothies to sweeten more bitter or sour fruits.

Apples are a highly sprayed crop in the United States, so it's important to buy organic apple juice from organic U.S. grown apples to avoid chemical exposure.

Applesauce

Fruit sauces such as applesauce contain all of the fiber of the fruit and most of the antioxidants. They add flavor and texture to smoothies and are a good way to meet our daily goal for intake of fruits and vegetables. Look for products with no added sugar or food coloring. Food colors, especially red dye #40, have been linked to ADHD and other hyperactivity disorders in children.

Apricots

Fresh, frozen, canned, or liquid apricot juice adds texture and sweetness to smoothies. Apricots contain beta-carotene, a potent antioxidant that prevents the buildup of plaque deposits in the arteries, protects the eyes from sun damage, and deactivates free radicals that, if left unchecked, accelerate the aging process and increase the risk of cancer. In addition, when the body is low on vitamin A, it will convert beta-carotene into vitamin A, which is vital for good vision and for keeping the eyes lubricated. Those at risk of dry eyes, such as contact-lens wearers, should include apricots and other beta-carotene-rich foods such as cantaloupe in their diet. Apricots also contain significant levels of iron, which is necessary for the transportation of oxygen via red blood cells. Iron deficiency leads to anemia, characterized by pale skin, and thinning, undernourished hair.

Avocados

Use ripe avocados as a base for creamy recipes, adding liquid as needed to create the consistency desired. They contain healthy fats, and are a nice choice for those needing a healthy increase in calories without saturated fats. They also deliver healthy amounts of potassium, folic acid, vitamin E, oleic acid, and protein. Avocados are so rich in oleic acid that they contain a higher ratio of this monounsaturated fat than even olive oil. Oleic acid is a fatty acid that has been credited with some of the heart-protective and anticancer properties of the traditional Mediterranean diet.

Avocados are also one of the richest studied sources of glutathione, an antioxidant that is part of the glutathione peroxidase enzyme. This enzyme is used by cells to defend against damage caused by free radicals. In addition, the vitamin E in avocados enhances the anticancer effects of glutathione.

The ripe flesh of an avocado has the consistency of firm butter and a taste reminiscent of nuts. Peel and pit each avocado before blending.

Bananas

Bananas are a good source of pectin, pyroxidine (B_6), potassium, magnesium, and folate. The pectin in bananas is a soluble fiber that adds a nice texture to smoothies while simultaneously reducing the risk of heart disease and several types of cancer.

Bananas are one of the more palatable forms of potassium, an electrolyte that is easily depleted through exercise, diarrhea, or the use of diuretics. Potassium is often helpful for reducing cramping, and increasing dietary potassium has been linked to reduced risk for hypertension.

Add a few pieces of frozen banana to smoothies for a creamy, milkshake-textured drink. Fresh bananas add thickness and body to smoothies. Organic bananas are a healthier choice than nonorganic, as most imported bananas are shipped into the country bathed in pesticides to kill tarantulas and other pests.

Barley Malt Sweetener

Barley malt is a liquid sweetener made from sprouted barley that is thick, dark, and similar to honey in consistency. Add it to smoothies to give them a malted flavor.

Berries

Dark berries such as blackberries, raspberries, cherries, and blueberries are lower in sugar than many sweet fruits and contain concentrated heart-healthy antioxidants. The most highly sprayed fruits include cherries, strawberries, imported grapes, peaches, and raspberries. To avoid chemical herbicide and pesticide residue, buy only organic berries and wash all fruits carefully.

Black Tea

Tea is made by steeping the leaves or buds of the tea bush *Camellia sinensis* in hot water for a few minutes. Tea processing can include oxidation (fermentation), heating, or drying of the leaves, or the addition of other herbs, spices, or fruits. There are four types of true tea: black tea, oolong tea, green tea, and white tea.

Black tea contains flavonoids, which have been found to lower the risk for vascular problems such as heart attack, stroke, and varicose veins. Tea is a natural source of caffeine, theophylline, and antioxidants.

Blueberries

Fresh or frozen berries impart a beautiful purple hue to your drinks while adding concentrations of powerful antioxidants and phytochemicals such as anthocyanins, ellagic acid, catechins, and resveratrol.

Brown Rice Syrup

Brown rice syrup is a minimally processed, mild sweetener made from sprouted brown rice.

Cane Sugar

The common white granulated cane sugar sold in most groceries today is made from the juice of the *Saccharum officinarum* plant, which has been refined and bleached. Turbinado sugar, which is darker in color, less refined, and unbleached, is a more complex and flavorful alternative, and contains calcium, iron, and vitamins.

Brown sugar is generally made by combining white sugar and molasses. Molasses is made by boiling sugar syrup. Once the sugar syrup has been boiled down through several processes, it is considered *blackstrap molasses*. It contains significant amounts of vitamins and minerals. Blackstrap molasses is a source of calcium, magnesium, and iron.

Cantaloupe

Cantaloupe (*Cucumis melo*) melon contains beta-carotene, vitamin C, and potassium and is low in calories.

Carambola

The carambola (*Averrhoa carambola*) is a fruit that originated in Sri Lanka (Ceylon) and the Maluku islands (Moluccas) of the Indonesian archipelago. Also called star fruit, carambola contains oxalic acid in varying levels depending on the variety. The sweeter varieties have lower oxalic acid. This fruit is a good source of vitamin C, beta-carotene, and potassium.

Carbonated Water

Look for beverages that are carbonated with CO_2 instead of phosphorous or phosphoric acid. Carbon dioxide is a gas that our bodies can break down, while phosphoric acid interferes with mineral absorption, which can lead to depletion of calcium in the bones. Desirable brands include San Faustino, San Pellegrino, and Perrier.

Cardamom

Elettaria cardamomum is a type of seed that has traditionally been used for treating indigestion, although it can also add a rich flavor to smoothies. It is available as whole pods or ground into powder.

Cassia

Cassia (Indonesian cinnamon) is also commonly called, and sometimes sold as, cinnamon.

Cherimoya

This fruit is a good source of vitamin C, riboflavin (B_2), and niacin (B_3).

Cherries

Cherries contain the potent antioxidant anthocyanins, as well as high levels of melatonin. Research has found a connection between low melatonin levels and heart attacks. Melatonin has also been shown to be important for functioning of the immune system, and has been shown to reduce inflammation by suppressing COX-2 in laboratory studies.

Chicory

Chicory has been used as a coffee alternative since the Middle Ages. Recently, extracts of chicory have been used as a base for natural sweeteners. Recently it was found that the root contains up to 20 percent inulin.

Chocolate

A study in the January 2006 issue of the journal Heart found that smokers who ate about 1½ ounces of dark chocolate daily had improved blood flow through their arteries.

Dark chocolate has a higher cocoa content than milk chocolate and less sugar. It is rich in antioxidants, which protect our bodies from the harmful effects of oxidation. See Cocoa for more information.

Cinnamon

Cinnamon contains a molecule with insulin-like properties that may help with type 2 diabetes. Studies have found that people with diabetes can lower their glucose levels if they take cinnamon. One study found that patients had significantly lower blood levels of glucose, triglycerides, and cholesterol after eating cinnamon for forty days. The flavor and scent come from cinnamic aldehyde or cinnamaldehyde, just one component of this rich, essential oil that also includes ethyl cinnamate, eugenol, beta-caryophyllene, linalool, and methyl chavicol.

Cocoa

Look for organic cocoa that is unsweetened and without food colors or preservatives. The darker chocolate contains higher levels of antioxidants than milk chocolate. Cocoa is rich in antioxidants and theobromine, a natural mood lifter.

Coconut

Components of coconut are currently being studied for their health properties and as an adjunct treatment for health conditions such as obesity. Coconut helps break down adipose tissue by increasing fat metabolism, serves as a treatment for arteriosclerosis (as it reduces cholesterol and triglyceride levels), assists in glycemic control (regulates insulin releases), eases stomach ulcers (antibacterial activity against H. *pylori*), and even fights cancer (influences tumor and host protein metabolism without stimulating tumor growth). Coconut also helps break down lipid-coated viruses, including measles, vercular stomatitis virus, herpes simplex virus, cytomegalovirus (CMV), and the influenza virus. It also fights the bacteria that cause staph infections and strep throat.

Coconut milk and coconut oil are widely available in stores and online. Prosperity Organic Foods makes a combination of flaxseed oil and coconut oil that is organic (see Resources section). The original formula and the sweet flavors of their Flax Spread add healthful oils to smoothies.

Coffee

Studies have shown that coffee is the main source of antioxidants for most Americans. Many fruits actually pack more antioxidant power per serving, but people consume them less frequently than coffee. The highest concentrations of antioxidants were found in dates, cranberries, and red grapes. The researchers found that both caffeinated and decaffeinated coffee appear to contain similar levels of antioxidants. Studies also show that the antioxidant chemicals in green and black tea are still present in decaffeinated alternatives.

For decaffeinated coffee, look for coffee that has been decaffeinated by the Swiss water process. It is much healthier than the common chemical process.

Cottage Cheese

Small-curd cottage cheese blends well into smoothies and makes an excellent source of protein for blender drinks.

Cucumber

A good source of electrolytes, cucumbers are fairly neutral in flavor and can be added to enhance the nutritional profile of many smoothie recipes without altering the flavor.

Dairy Products

Nonorganic dairy products in the United States have residue of synthetic bovine growth hormone (BGH), which is also known as recombinant bovine somatotropin (BST). Women and children are especially susceptible to health problems caused by hormones such as BGH in milk. Buy organic, as the USDA does not allow synthetic hormones in foods labeled "organic."

I also recommend fortified milk as it has a host of additional nutrients added to it, most commonly vitamins D and A, and sometimes vitamin E or calcium.

Dates

Dates contain fiber, folacin, and salicylates, which fight cancer and heart disease; trace minerals and calcium, which build bone density; and iron, which prevents fatigue and menstrual problems.

Date puree is the easiest way to sweeten smoothies with dates. Purchase whole, fresh, or dried dates, all of which are rich sources of fiber, potassium, and antioxidants. Puree them in a blender with water before adding them to any recipe.

Date sugar is a sweet powder made from ground dried dates.

Electrolytes

Electrolyte powders are high-quality, inexpensive sources of the electrolytes that are lost through sweat. Electrolyte liquids are also available. Replacing electrolytes is important for those who have been ill, for athletes, and for those recovering from dehydration.

Figs

Figs add sweetness and nutritional value to smoothies. They contain notable amounts of protein, calcium, magnesium, phosphorus, and potassium. Figs also contain ficin, a protein-breaking enzyme similar to papain in papayas and bromelin in fresh pineapple. Ficin also has some laxative effects. Dried figs can be stored in the refrigerator or at room temperature; however, fresh figs should always be refrigerated. Dried figs may keep for several weeks.

Fish Oil

Udòs Oil and Coromega are two highly recommended companies that make tasty flavored fish oil products. Fish oils are extremely important sources of EFAs, which help our cells stay hydrated when they absorb water.

Flaxseed

Flaxseeds contain soluble fiber, omega-3 fatty acids, and magnesium. Flaxseeds should be ground before using for better digestion and to release the beneficial oils inside the shells. Freeze for long-term storage. Flaxseed oil can be used raw in smoothies.

Folic Acid

Folic acid supplementation has been found to reduce incidence of depression, anxiety, birth defects, and fatigue syndromes. Liquid folic acid is widely available and inexpensive. It is water soluble, which means it is nontoxic as your body will only absorb what it needs.

Fruit Sauces

Applesauce and other whole-fruit sauces contain soluble fibers such as pectin, which help stabilize blood sugar levels and reduce cholesterol levels.

Ginger

The main medicinal compounds in ginger are phenolic compounds such as gingerols and shogaols, and sesquiterpenes such as zingiberene. These and other compounds are extracts found in ginger oleoresin. The main pungent flavor chemicals are the gingerols, which are not volatile. It is thought to be an anti-inflammatory and an antioxidant, which boost the immune system and naturally increase the body's energy levels.

Ginger Ale

Ginger ale is a tasty, noncaffeinated beverage and a soothing digestive aid.

Grapefruit

Grapefruit of all varieties is high in antioxidants, but recent studies have found that red grapefruit is even more effective in reducing cholesterol levels. Fresh grapefruit can be added to smoothies as a daily part of a cholesterol-reduction program.

Grapefruit is derived from a bitter citrus fruit known as the pomelo, which was cross-pollinated with the orange to make it sweeter; however, the grapefruit was not recognized as a distinct species of citrus fruit until the nineteenth century. The tangy fruit increases metabolism, which is why it is often eaten after breakfast and used for body detoxification.

Grapefruit contains pectin, an acid shown in animal studies to reduce LDL cholesterol and add appreciable amounts of glutathione, an amino acid compound that has been shown in animal studies to help reduce atherosclerosis (narrowing and hardening of the arteries). Pink and red grapefruit have higher concentrations of the antioxidant pigments beta-carotene and lycopene. Both of these carotenoids have cancer-protective effects. The redder the fruit, the more it contains.

Grapefruit also offers potassium, which lowers high blood pressure; pectin, which lowers cholesterol levels; vitamin C, which helps stabilize unstable plaque lesions in arteries; glutathione, the nutrient used by the liver for detoxification; folate, which detoxifies homocysteine and prevents birth defects; and boatloads of flavanoids including terpenes, D-limonene, and coumarins, which help prevent cancer. Pink grapefruit is also a source of two carotenes, beta-carotene and beta-cryptoxanthin.

The flavanoid naringenin, found only in grapefruit, inhibits several of the liver enzymes responsible for drug metabolism. If you take calcium channel blockers, cyclosporine, or a benzodiazepine, check with your physician or pharmacist before adding grapefruit to your smoothies. Naringenin also prolongs the length of time that caffeine remains in the blood.

Grapes

Grapes, grape juice, and wine all contain the flavanoid resveratrol, which is found in grape skins. Flavanols are naturally occurring, healthful phytochemicals found in varying levels in all fruits and vegetables. Apples, grapes, berries, and tea have particularly high levels.

Green Tea

Green tea may help prevent prostate cancer. Green tea contains catechins—chemicals that may inhibit a key molecule involved in the development of prostate cancer. Look for powdered green tea products with high levels of catechins, such as TeaTech, which has eight times the antioxidants of most tea. Green teas have more antioxidants than do black or oolong varieties.

Guava

Guava is a fruit that should be eaten quickly once ripe as they stay good for only about two days. You can refrigerate them for a short period, but they get tough and become significantly less appetizing. Guava nectar is widely available in grocery stores and the best way to purchase guava for smoothies.

Hemp Seeds

Hemp seeds are an excellent source of essential fatty acids and provide protein to smoothies.

Herbal Tea

Herbal tea refers to infusions made from herbs such as rose hips, chamomile, and mint leaves. Herbal teas are also known as tisanes.

Honey

Raw, unpasteurized honey has not been heat-treated and is believed to contain natural antibacterial agents. It is sold in either liquid or dry crystallized form. Babies should not be fed honey, as their gastrointestinal tracts are not fully formed until six months to one year of age. They are at risk for food poisoning from honey until after their first year.

Ice Cream

The highest quality ice cream contains only organic milk (or alternative milk such as soymilk or rice milk), and has no hydrogenated oils, synthetic food coloring, or other additives.

Inulin-FOS

Inulin-FOS (FructoOligoSaccharide) is a soluble fiber and promotes beneficial intestinal bacterial growth. For this reason, it

is often added to yogurt and other products that have been in-
oculated with beneficial microflora.

Just Like Sugar™

This alternative sweetener is made from chicory root, orange
peel, and vitamin C. Unlike other natural sweeteners on the
market, which have a characteristic intense sweet and bitter
licorice aftertaste, Just Like Sugar™ has a proprietary formula-
tion that tastes clean, smooth, and sweet. It does not leave an
aftertaste.

Kiwifruit

Kiwifruit is an excellent source of vitamin C, potassium, and dietary fiber and is also a good source of vitamin E, folate, magnesium, copper, and lutein.

Kumquats

These sweet-and-sour fruits add a bright high note to smoothies. Nutritionally they offer a healthy dose of calcium, potassium, and vitamin C.

Lecithin

Lecithin is a dietary source of choline, a promising nutrient
for improving memory. Choline is needed to produce acetylcholine, a neurotransmitter, and is also a component of cell
membranes and myelin, the insulating sheath around the
nerves. Choline is essential for proper brain development in
infants and children. Lecithin is a special type of fat called a
phospholipid; its chemical name is phosphatidylcholine. Lecithin liquid and granules, made from soybeans, can be purchased
and added to smoothies. Wheat germ and peanut butter are natural sources of lecithin.

Lemons

Lemons have natural plant chemicals (phytochemicals) called
monoterpenes in their skin that both protect against cells be-

coming cancerous and help fight existing cancers. Eat only organic lemons, as commercial citrus may have been sprayed with antifungal chemicals to prevent storage rot. (They may also be dyed to heighten the color and waxed with a vegetable-derived wax to improve the appearance.)

Licorice

Licorice root is an herb that has been used for thousands of years in Eastern cultures. Its medicinally active component is glycyrrhizin, which breaks down into glycyrrhetinic acid, or GA. GA has anti-inflammatory properties that may aid in the relief of arthritis pain. Licorice is also used to boost immune function and protect the liver from chemical toxins.

Those with high blood pressure should avoid licorice, as it can raise blood pressure when used frequently at high doses. Deglycyrrhized licorice is safe for those with elevated blood pressure and is widely available in powder form.

Limes

Limes, like lemons, have natural plant chemicals (phytochemicals) called monoterpenes in their skin that both protect against cells becoming cancerous and help fight existing cancers. Purchase only the organic variety.

Luo Han Guo Fruit

Luo han guo (or lo han) is a very sweet fruit grown in China. Extracts of luo han guo are now being marketed as a sweetener. The amounts normally used are so small that luo han guo is not likely to have an appreciable effect on human physiology. Mogrosides, which are water-soluble molecules extracted from the luo han guo fruit, offer a pleasant, sweet taste without elevating blood sugar. Luo han guo mogrosides are also up to 250 times sweeter than sugar, making this an excellent smoothie sweetener substitute.

Lychees

Lychees are delicious and rich in vitamin C. They are available in tropical areas and also sold in cans throughout the United States.

Malted Milk Powder

Plain malted milk powder is made from dry powdered milk and malt powder (ground dried sprouted barley). It dissolves well in smoothies and adds protein as well as B vitamins to drinks.

Maltitol

Malitol is a popular sugar alcohol. It does not raise blood-sugar levels the way regular table sugar does because it is not absorbed by the body. It is a sugar substitute that is safe for diabetics to use, as it does not raise blood sugar levels, but it can cause digestive distress in large quantities.

Mangoes

Mangoes are an excellent source of beta-carotene and vitamin C. Peel them and slice the flesh away from the pit. Store the mango flesh in a plastic bag in the freezer. Mango nectar, frozen mango slices, mango puree, and mango juice are all widely available and make great smoothie ingredients.

Mangosteens

A tropical fruit currently being studied for its health benefits. The juice is now widely available.

Maple Syrup

The syrup made from the boiled-down sap of sugar maple trees is sweet and contains more minerals than cane sugar. The highest quality maple syrup is pure, which means it is 100 percent sap syrup with no cane sugar or corn syrup added. USDA grade B maple syrup is darker, has a stronger flavor, and may contain more minerals than grade A.

Milk Substitutes

Milk made from grains such as oat milk and rice milk are good liquid bases for smoothies. Flavored grain milks can come in plain, vanilla, chocolate, and other flavors. Neither cow's milk nor grain milk is considered an acceptable alternative for breast-feeding or specially designed infant formula.

Mineral Water

Mineral water contains naturally occurring minerals and electrolytes. Look for mineral water in glass bottles, such as Perrier, San Pellegrino, or San Faustino. The latter is the "Calcium Water"; one glass of San Faustino provides 10 percent of the adult RDA for calcium. Adding mineral water to a smoothie adds a clean water source to help you hydrate with minerals that aid in the absorption of the water. They are also a healthy way to add carbonation to a drink. Avoid drinks that are carbonated with phosphoric acid or phosphorous, as this mineral competes for the binding sites on your cells with minerals such as calcium, causing nutrient deficiencies.

Mint

Mint was originally used as a medicinal herb to treat stomachaches and chest pains. During the Middle Ages, powdered mint leaves were used to whiten teeth. Mint tea is a strong diuretic.

Nectars

Thick juices containing fruit fiber are known as nectars and are becoming very popular as health drinks and as smoothie ingredients.

Nonfat Dry Milk Powder

This powder is sold in almost all grocery stores. It reconstitutes easily, so it blends quickly with other smoothie ingredients.

Each tablespoon of powder contains more than a gram of protein. Try to buy the organic variety to avoid added hormones.

Nutmeg

Nutmeg is a highly valued spice indigenous to the Maluku Islands, near Indonesia. It is not generally known that nutmeg is actually the kernel of the apricot-like fruit of the tree *Myristica fragrans*, and that it is enclosed in a hard seed case covered with a soft membranous coat that is used to create the spice mace.

Nutritional Yeast

Nutritional yeast (*Saccharomyces cerevisiae*) is not to be mistaken with the equally healthy but bitter brewer's yeast. Nutritional yeast is grown specifically for its nutritive value and is widely available at natural food stores. It contains B vitamins and tastes great on popcorn as well as in smoothies.

Nuts

Nuts contain tocopherols, a group of fat-soluble molecules that help protect the immune and cardiovascular systems. Nuts are also high in arginine, polyphenols, vitamin E, unsaturated fat, and fiber. These nutrients protect the heart from disease.

All nuts can be ground into butters, which serve as healthy vegetarian protein sources. Buy nut butters that are free of hydrogenated oils, which increase the risk of cardiovascular disease.

Oranges

Oranges contain high levels of folate and vitamin C. Unless they are certified as organically grown, commercial citrus may have been sprayed with anti-fungal chemicals to prevent storage rot. They may also be dyed to heighten the color and coated with a vegetable-derived wax to heighten their appearance.

Papayas

One serving of papaya will meet about 20 percent of an adult's daily folate needs and 75 percent of the daily vitamin C requirement.

Passionfruit

The passionfruit *Passiflora edulis* is native to an area that stretches from southern Brazil to northern Argentina. Passionfruits have the third highest potassium level of any domestic fruit. They also have useful amounts of beta-carotene.

Peaches

The ancestral species *Prunus persica*, which gave rise to both the almond and the peach, was probably native to Central Asia. One medium peach supplies about 5 percent of an adult's minimum daily niacin (B_3) requirement. Fresh and canned peaches have about the same amount of carotenoids.

Peanut Butter

Peanut butter is simply ground peanuts with a little salt. Some stores have nut grinders so you can make your own fresh peanut butter, and there are many high-quality brands available, such as Kettle and Maranatha, that are as pure as they come. Peanuts grow in moist, hot places and some have a tendency to develop a fungal infection that produces a toxin called aflatoxin. Many peanut butter manufacturers now test for aflatoxins to be sure their products are free from contamination. Peanut butter is an excellent source of protein.

Pectin

Pectin, extracted from fruits such as apples, plums, gooseberries, and oranges, is sold as a thickening agent and is used in food products such as yogurt. Pectin helps lower cholesterol and reduce hardening of the arteries.

Persimmons

Persimmons are an excellent source of vitamin C, depending on the variety. Persimmons also contain lycopene, a carotenoid protective against prostate cancer.

Pineapples

Most pineapple varieties are a good source of vitamin C (a typical serving has around 13 mg, about 20 percent of the recommend daily intake for an adult). Canned pineapple loses a third of its vitamin C content in processing, but it still contains a useful amount. Pineapples contain the enzyme bromelain, which scientists suspect may reduce the synthesis of inflammatory substances in the body.

Plums

Plums provide potassium, fiber, vitamin K, and trace levels of magnesium, iron, and vitamin C. Plums also have useful levels of riboflavin (B_2), with two medium plums providing about a sixteenth of an adult's recommended daily intake, and are a fairly good source of vitamin C. They also contain high levels of phenolic compounds and antioxidants that may protect against age-related macular degeneration and cataracts.

Pomegranates

Pomegranates, pomegranate juice, and pomegranate extracts are now available year-round in the United States. A rich source of vitamin C, folic acid, and antioxidants, pomegranates are also high in hydrosolubale tannins, an antioxidant polyphenol responsible for free-radical scavenging.

In several clinical trials, the juice of the pomegranate has been found effective in reducing the risk of heart disease. Tannins have been identified as the primary components responsible for the reduction of oxidative states, which lead to heart disease.

Protein Powders

Protein shakes are easier to digest than solid food, so they are a good choice when you don't have time to stop for a meal or when you are recovering from an illness.

- **Soy protein powder** Soy foods that are not organic have been genetically engineered to have a higher resistance to specific herbicides, and have high residue levels of these carcinogenic chemicals. Buy organic to avoid these agricultural chemicals and GMOs. Vanilla soy powders are often favored over plain, as plain soy often has a beany flavor.

- **Whey protein powder** Whey is the protein component of dairy. As long as you are not sensitive or allergic to dairy, whey is a great choice for you. It contains glutathione, a powerful detoxifier, and is generally well absorbed in the digestive system. It mixes well with dairy-based drinks and adds a creamy texture.

- **Rice protein powder** For those with allergies, rice is often the best choice, as it has the least allergenic potential of all protein powders. It has a mild flavor, and mixes better with drinks that have grains, as it may not dissolve completely.

- **Pea protein powder** Pea-based protein powder contains protein as well as fiber, so it packs even more of a nutritional punch. It's a wonderful alternative to the more common protein supplements, as it digests easily and has low allergenic potential.

Pumpkin

Pumpkin seeds are the best vegetarian source of zinc, with 7 mg in every 3 ounces—that is half of the daily recommended intake. Pumpkin puree can be bought in a can and added to smoothies. You can also buy a whole pumpkin, cook it, remove the pulp, and use the pulp in a smoothie. Either way, it is an exceptional source of carotenoids, which are powerful protectors from the sun's damaging rays and environmental toxins.

Psyllium

Psyllium husk powder is available at many grocery and health food stores. It is a bulking agent that thickens and emulsifies smoothies, which is helpful when making cold drinks with a high water content. The psyllium helps keep the ingredients from separating and the smoothie creamier longer. Psyllium is a gentle bulk-forming laxative.

Raspberries

Fresh or frozen raspberries have many medicinal properties, such as protecting against oxidative damage, helping to reduce cholesterol levels, stabilizing blood sugar levels, and providing support to the immune system.

Rice Milk

Rice is one of the least allergenic foods there is and for this reason, rice milk is often used as an alternative to dairy products. Like soymilk, it is available in plain or vanilla. Rice milk is a good base for many smoothies, as it does not add a strong flavor and won't overpower the other ingredients.

Rooibos Tea

Red tea may also refer to rooibos tea, an increasingly popular South African tisane.

Soybean Products

Soybeans contain naturally occurring phytochemicals such as the isoflavones daidzein, genistein, and glycitein. Soy foods, such as tofu and soymilk, have been found to help reduce blood cholesterol levels. Soy foods also contain iron, which helps deliver oxygen throughout the body. Since 39 percent of Americans are not getting enough iron, it's a good idea to incorporate one serving of a soy product in your diet daily. Add soy protein powder to smoothies for a protein boost. However, if you have low thyroid production or if you take thyroid medication, you should avoid soy products as they interfere with absorption of thyroid hormones.

Sparkling Water

Sparkling water in glass bottles, such as San Faustino, San Pellegrino, and Perrier, are carbonated with CO_2, which is natural and safe. Other types of carbonation, such as those that incorporate phosphoric acid or phosphorus, interfere with mineral absorption and should therefore be avoided. Also, avoid water in plastic bottles as plastic particles can migrate into the water, leading to the ingestion of unhealthy endocrine-disrupting substances.

Star Fruit

Star fruit is an excellent source of vitamin C and fiber. See *Carambola*.

Stevia

Stevia is a noncaloric sweetener made from an herb native to South America. It is safe for diabetics and appears to be nontoxic.

Strawberries

Strawberries have high quantities of vitamin C; five strawberries provide more than half the daily requirement for an adult. The phytonutrient phenols most abundant in strawberries are anthocyanins and ellagitannins. The anthocyanins help to prevent oxidative damage from free radicals in the body. The phenol compounds help protect the heart and fight inflammation.

Sugar

Refined sugar is not recommended in smoothies, as most are sweetened naturally. If you find that a sweetener is required and you don't have any natural sweeteners about, use turbinado or raw sugar in moderation.

Tangerines

Tangerines are a good source of beta-carotene—in fact, they rank number 5 in the list of top sources from commercial fruit. They are also a very good source of vitamin C: one tangerine provides almost half an adult's daily requirement. Unless they are certified organically grown, commercial citrus may have been sprayed with antifungal chemicals to prevent storage rot. (They may also be dyed to heighten the color and coated with a vegetable-derived wax to improve the appearance.)

Tea

There are many types of exotic and healthful teas available today. Experiment until you find the teas that you like best, brew them, and store the prepared tea for up to four days in the refrigerator in a glass pitcher. You will then have tea on hand to add to smoothies on a whim.

Try traditional *Camellia sinensis* teas in white, green, oolong (Chinese tea between green and black in oxidation), or black. White, green, oolong, then black is the approximate order from most to least healthful, as darker teas have been oxidized longer and have fewer antioxidants. American chai tea adds a combination of spices, including cloves, cinnamon, nutmeg, ginger, cardamom, and/or pepper. Other interesting teas include yerba mate, a traditional South American infusion; rooibos or red tea, which is a caffeine-free tisane from South Africa; and chamomile, peppermint, passionfruit (useful for some with insomnia), anise, licorice, genmaicha, mugicha (Japanese barley tea), ginger, lemongrass, and rose hip teas.

Tofu

Soybean curd, or tofu, is neutral in flavor and becomes smooth and creamy when added to smoothies. It is a great protein source and imparts all of the health benefits of the soybean, including fiber and isoflavones such as genestein and daidzein. Use silken tofu when possible, which is a creamy tofu sold in the aseptic boxes. Look for the word *organic* on the box.

Turbinado Sugar

Unrefined evaporated cane juice is also known as turbinado sugar. It is less processed than white cane sugar, has not been treated with bleach, and contains naturally occurring minerals from sugarcane. Needless to say it's delicious, but high in calories, so use sparingly.

Vanilla

The vanilla bean comes from the pod of the tropical Mexican orchid vine *Vanilla planifolia* (v. *fragrans*). Real vanilla extract, not to be confused with artificial vanilla, has a rich flavor that enhances the sweet flavors already in a smoothie, giving it depth and richness. Artificial vanilla is a poor imitation of true vanilla as it lacks the quality of the natural vanilla flavor that develops during the curing of the beans, when glucosides are converted to vanillic aldehyde or vanillin. Vanilla extract in an alcohol or glycerin base can be found in grocery stores, and many specialty stores carry vanilla beans. The seeds or soft center from the beans can be scraped out and added to smoothies.

Vitamin C

Vitamin C powder dissolves well in smoothies and has just slight citrus flavor, so it hides well in many different types of smoothies. It is an important antioxidant that supports the immune system and helps protect the body from environmental toxins. Vitamin C powder is available in a wide range of flavors for fizzy, naturally flavored drinks that make healthy soda pop alternatives and smoothie additions.

Water

Buy either bottled water in glass bottles or water filtered with an activated, solid-carbon filter in order to avoid contaminants.

Watermelon

Watermelon contains electrolytes, vitamin C, and carotenoids. It is also a good source of glutathione, a powerful antioxidant and anticarcinogen. Watermelons contain an amino acid called citrulline that has diuretic properties, good for people who retain water. Best of all, watermelons have 60 percent more of the antioxidant lycopene than raw tomatoes.

Wheat Germ

Wheat germ contains vitamin E, B vitamins, calcium, iron, potassium, and selenium and is also an excellent source of iron, magnesium, zinc, and niacin. As far as smoothie ingredients go, it is one of the best sources of cysteine, an amino acid that plays a major role in the detoxification of metals and environmental toxins from our bodies. Cysteine is also an antimucagenic, which means it helps break down mucus and flush it from our systems.

Coenzyme Q_{10} (CoQ10) deficiency results in a reduced ability to produce the enzymes needed to break down body fat. Increasing CoQ10 in supplement or whole-food form can restore the enzymatic action in fat cells, which allows release of stored fat. Toasted wheat germ is the perfect CoQ10-containing food to add to smoothies as it blends well, has very little taste, and almost disappears in a creamy drink.

Xylitol

Xylitol, a naturally occurring polyol, also called wood sugar or birch sugar, is sweet and cool in the mouth. It can be extracted from birch, raspberries, plums, and corn and is primarily produced in China.

Xylitol is as sweet as sugar, but has 40 percent less calories than cane sugar products. It has been heavily used in Japan since the early 1970s with no ill effects. Xylitol is metabolized differently from a conventional sugar and does not cause or contribute to tooth decay. In fact, studies have established that it inhibits the bacteria responsible for tooth decay. Xylitol, like most sugar alcohols, can have a mild laxative effect at high doses. It has no known toxicity, though; people have consumed as much as 400 grams daily for long periods with no apparent ill effects.

Yogurt

Yogurt is fermented milk that was once associated with grounded spirituality and inspiration. In the sixteenth century, it was used to treat depression, and a limited diet consisting mostly of yogurt is thought to be the reason some Balkan people live more than a hundred years. Read product labels to be sure the yogurt you buy is organic and free of synthetic sweeteners, food colorings, and corn syrup.

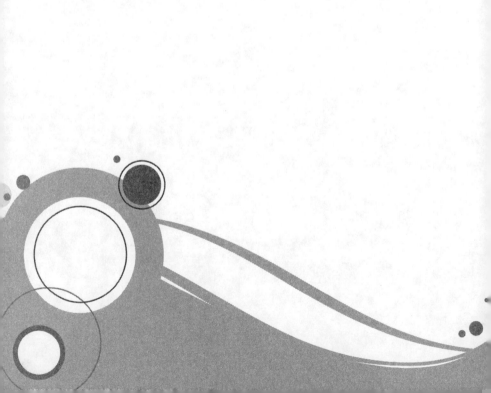

resources

Supplements for Smoothies

Alacer Corp.
Foothill Ranch, CA 92610
www.alacercorp.com

This is the famous maker of the powdered vitamin C product (Emergen-C) and the electrolyte powder (Electro-Mix) that can be added to smoothies.

Coromega Company
2460 Coral Street
Vista, CA 92081
Toll Free: 877-275-3725
Consumer Questions: support@coromega.com

This is the company that makes the orange-flavored fish oil that kids and adults love.

Natural Calm
Peter Gillham's Natural Vitality
4867 Fountain Avenue
Los Angeles, CA 90029
www.petergillham.com

Powdered magnesium products such as Calm and Mama Calm.

Ingredients for Smoothies

Cascadian Farm
55749 State Route 20
Rockport, WA 98283
www.cascadianfarm.com

They offer whole frozen fruit and concentrate, including blueberries, straw-berries, raspberries, sliced peaches, cherries, harvest berries, blackberries, frozen fruit; orange, grape, apple, lemonade, raspberry, cranberry fruit con-centrate. Cascadian Farm bottled and frozen juices are high quality, organic, and consistently sweet and fresh. Their products are widely available.

Dagoba
Toll Free: 877-992-4626 (877-99-CHOCO)
Fax Toll Free: 877-912-4626

They make organic chocolate bars and cocoa powder.

Eden Foods
701 Tecumseh Road
Clinton, MI 49236
Phone: 888-424-3336

Eden products are available in most grocery stores.

ESHA Research Inc.
Scott Hadsall
Phone: 800-659-3742
www.ESHA.com

This is the company that makes the software used to create the nutrition facts food labels (analysis) throughout this book. It can also be purchased for home use to analyze your diet or that of your family.

Happy Honu Farm
Joan and Tom Lamont
Phone: 808-329-0718

Offers tropical canned goods, jams. Happy Honu Farm grows organic tropical fruit, then cans and ships. They make jellies and marmalades that add a rich flavor to smoothies.

Just Like Sugar, Inc.
Las Vegas, NV 89119
Phone: 866-547-8417

This company offers the delicious sugar substitute Just Like Sugar, made from chicory, orange peel, and vitamin C, which is safe for diabetics. It actually does taste just like sugar, dissolves well in smoothies, and you can bake with it. I love this product! It's sold in Whole Foods markets, natural foods markets, and many grocery stores.

Kanalani Ohana Farm
Colehour and Melanie Bondera
P.O. Box 861
Honaunau, HI 96726
Phone: 808-328-0296
www.kanalanifarm.org
colemel@efn.org

This organic farm has a coffee CSA (Community Supported Agriculture) program. You can sign up for a period of time and they will send you fresh organic coffee on a regular basis.

Kuaiwi Farm
Una Greenaway
P.O. Box 999
Captain Cook, HI 96704
Phone: 808-328-8888
www.kuaiwifarm.com

This little farm grows organic coffee and macadamia nuts. They make a certified organic raw macadamia nut butter that is excellent in smoothies. These are quality farmers with fresh products. They will ship.

Pacific Natural Foods
19480 SW 97th Avenue
Tualatin, OR 97602
Phone: 503-692-9666
www.pacificfoods.com

This company makes organic soy beverages as well as nut and grain beverages. They are widely available through mainstream grocery stores.

Prosperity Organic Foods
Cygnia Rapp
Hailey, ID 83333
www.prosperityorganicfoods.com

Organic Coconut Flax Butter is a creamy vegan product made from extra-virgin coconut oil and organic flaxseed oil. Organic Coconut Flax Butter is rich in healthful lauric and essential fatty acids, and is available in flavors that work well for smoothies, such as the Original and Sweet Orange. Contact Prosperity Organic Foods at 208-309-2754 for mail-order services.

San Faustino
Phone: 866-537-7349

This mineral water contains medicinal quantities of calcium, tastes great, and is a good liquid base for smoothies.

TeaTech
TeaTech.com

The makers of high-antioxidant green tea powder that dissolves in water.

Udòs Oil
www.udoerasmus.com

The makers of high-quality organic omega oil blends, greens, digestive enzymes, and probiotics.

Vitasoy USA Inc.
One New England Way
Ayer, MA 01432
Phone: 800-848-1769
Vitasoy-usa.com

Vitasoy makes soy beverages, such as their Classic Original, Vanilla Delight, Creamy Original, Smooth Vanilla, Lite Original, Lite Vanilla, Green Tea Soymilk, and Unsweetened Original.

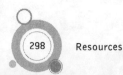

index

More Great Smoothie Recipes from
Daniella Chace

Blend Your Way to Better Health!

Featuring tantalizing smoothies based on creative combinations of antioxidant-rich fruits, flavorful extracts, and natural sweeteners, *Smoothies for Life!* includes information for adding revitalizing herbs such as ginkgo, echinacea, goldenseal, and kava! Learn how you can:

- Build athletic endurance with Tropical Elixir
- Lose weight with Peachy Almond Freeze
- Reduce stress with Ginseng Soother
- Detoxify your body with Watermelon Cooler
- And much more!

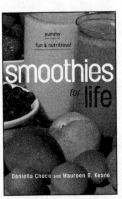

Smoothies for Life!
978-0-7615-1340-7
$14.95 paper (Canada: $22.95)

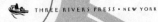

THREE RIVERS PRESS • NEW YORK

Available from Three Rivers Press wherever books are sold.